'Rarely has a book made such a difference to me than this one. When I was having tests and assessments which resulted in a dementia diagnosis, this book was my supporting prop. It removed my fear and gave me answers to the questions I confronted. An essential book for all.'

– Keith Oliver, Alzheimer's Society Ambassador and KMPT NHS Dementia Envoy

'This "pocket"-sized guide packs a full-sized punch. It answers in clear terms all the important questions about dementia. Dispels much of the stigma and misunderstanding associated with the disease. Offers practical guidance and support, and will be especially valuable to those who are carers.'

– Angela Rippon, CBE

'If you are struggling with the puzzling behaviours of an older relative, neighbour or one of your patients or clients who you think may have dementia, this factual and plainly written guide is the perfect introduction, updated to provide really practical current advice.'

– Baroness Elaine Murphy, Vice President of the Alzheimer's Society

'This is the book I wish I'd had while accompanying my mother on her long dementia journey. The information we were desperate for is here, the questions we asked are answered – clearly, simply and with some great practical tips. It could make all the difference to caregivers.'

– Sally Magnusson, author of Where Memories Go: Why Dementia Changes Everything *and founder of the charity Playlist for Life*

of related interest

Dementia – Support for Family and Friends
Dave Pulsford and Rachel Thompson
ISBN 978 1 84905 243 6
eISBN 978 0 85700 504 5

Can I tell you about Dementia?
A guide for family, friends and carers
Jude Welton
Illustrated by Jane Telford
ISBN 978 1 84905 297 9
eISBN 978 0 85700 634 9

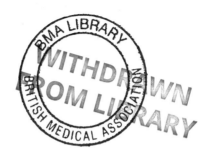

A Pocket Guide to Understanding Alzheimer's Disease and Other Dementias

Second Edition

Dr James Warner and Dr Nori Graham

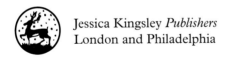

Jessica Kingsley *Publishers*
London and Philadelphia

First edition published in 2009 by Family Doctor Publications
This edition published in 2018
by Jessica Kingsley Publishers
73 Collier Street
London N1 9BE, UK
and
400 Market Street, Suite 400
Philadelphia, PA 19106, USA

www.jkp.com

Library of Congress Cataloging in Publication Data
Names: Warner, James (James Peregrine William), 1962- author.
Title: A pocket guide to understanding Alzheimer's disease and other
    dementias / Dr. James Warner and Dr. Nori Graham.
Description: Second edition. | London ; Philadelphia : Jessica Kingsley
    Publishers, 2018. | Revised edition of: Understanding Alzheimer's disease
    and other dementias / by Nori Graham and James Warner. ISBN 9781903474617.
    Family Doctor Publications, 2009. | Includes index.
Identifiers: LCCN 2017047866 | ISBN 9781785924583 (alk. paper)
Subjects: LCSH: Alzheimer's disease. | Dementia.
Classification: LCC RC523 .W359 2018 | DDC 616.8/311--dc23 LC record available
at https://lccn.loc.gov/2017047866

British Library Cataloguing in Publication Data
A CIP catalogue record for this book is available from the British Library

ISBN 978 1 78592 458 3
eISBN 978 1 78450 835 7

Printed and bound in China

Important Notice

This information is intended not as a substitute for personal medical advice but as a supplement to that advice for the patient who wishes to understand more about his or her condition.

Before taking any form of treatment *you should always consult your medical practitioner*. In particular (without limit), you should note that advances in medical science occur rapidly and some of the information about drugs and treatment may very soon be out of date.

About the Authors

Dr James Warner BSc, MBBS, MD, MRCP, FRCPsych is a consultant in old age psychiatry in Central North West London Foundation NHS Trust and Medical Director of Halcyon Doctors. He works in teams providing assessment and treatment of older people with mental illness and dementia. Dr Warner's academic interests include teaching, evidence-based psychiatry and research into dementia. He has contributed to over 100 scientific papers, several books and book chapters. Dr Warner was chair of the Faculty of Old Age Psychiatry at the Royal College of Psychiatrists from 2012 to 2016 and is National Advisor at the Care Quality Commission.

Dr Nori Graham BM, BCh, FRCPsych (Hon), DUniv is Emeritus Consultant in the Psychiatry of Old Age at the Royal Free Hospital, where she was responsible for many years for a community-oriented multidisciplinary service for older people with mental illness. She was the National Chairman of the Alzheimer's Society for England from 1987 to 1994, and Chairman of Alzheimer's Disease International (ADI), the umbrella organisation of national Alzheimer associations worldwide, from 1996 to 2002. She is now Vice-President of the Alzheimer's Society, England, and Honorary Vice-President of ADI. Currently she is a non-executive director for Residential Care Services of Care UK. In 1996, she was awarded an honorary doctorate for public services by the Open University.

Acknowledgements

We wish to thank Rachid Rhouzzal, a social worker in the Royal Borough of Kensington and Chelsea, for providing up-to-date information on resources and benefits.

We also thank Professor John O'Brien and Dr Elijah Mak of Cambridge University for MRI images.

Contents

1
Introduction

WHO IS THIS BOOK FOR?

- I think my memory is going?
- I have a relative or friend who has started behaving oddly?
- What is Alzheimer's disease?
- Is Alzheimer's disease the same as dementia?
- What can I do to stop getting dementia?

If these are the sorts of questions that you are asking yourself, this book is for you. Dementia is a disease of the brain. First, we define dementia before going on to list the symptoms. This chapter helps you decide whether you, a member of your family or a friend may have dementia.

Next, we discuss treatment and how to get help, and after that we give some tips on how to make the best of life if you or a loved one is found to have dementia. Then we consider how future developments may change the outlook for people with dementia, and describe some common questions and give some answers. Finally, we describe how the brain works. Some of that chapter is a bit technical, so you may decide to skip it.

There is a lot of myth and misinformation about dementia. This book is intended for anyone who has dementia or may be worried that they or their family and friends have dementia.

This book is also invaluable for people who live or work with someone with dementia.

We hope that by reading this book you will have a better understanding of what causes the illness and how it is diagnosed and treated.

WHAT IS DEMENTIA?

'Dementia' is a term used to describe any condition where a variety of different brain functions such as memory, thinking, recognition, language, planning and personality deteriorate over time.

Dementia is not part of normal ageing. Everyone gets more forgetful as they get older; that does not mean that they have dementia. The most common type of dementia is Alzheimer's disease, but there are several other types.

WHO GETS DEMENTIA?

Dementia is common. It is estimated that there are over three-quarters of a million people with dementia in the UK and this number is rising. As people get older the risk of dementia increases rapidly. It is estimated that one in five people aged over 80 years has some type of dementia.

Dementia can affect anyone. Prominent people such as Ronald Reagan, Harold Wilson, Margaret Thatcher, Iris Murdoch, Terry Pratchett and many other well-known names from all walks of life have developed dementia. It is a global problem, occurring in all ethnic groups and all social classes. No one is immune.

It is important to recognise when someone may have dementia. A swift and accurate diagnosis is important while people can still plan their lives and have a say in their treatment. Getting a diagnosis is also helpful to explain why someone isn't getting on as well as they used to and it ensures that they get the necessary help. It is also reassuring to be told if you don't have dementia.

FACTS AND FIGURES ABOUT DEMENTIA

Dementia is common; about 1 in every 90 people in the UK has dementia. In 2017, it was estimated that there were over 750,000 people in the UK with dementia and this will rise to over one million by 2030.

Dementia is rare below the age of 65, but can occur in people as young as 30. About 1 in 20 people over the age of 65 has dementia, rising to about one in five people aged over 80. Two-thirds of people with dementia live at home, and over three-quarters of people living in care homes have dementia.

Dementia is becoming more common because the biggest risk factor for dementia is getting older, and people are living longer. However, the number of new cases of dementia per 1000 of the population is reducing, mainly because of better general health. One in three people with dementia never get the condition diagnosed.

People who develop dementia often live for many years with the condition. Nearly everyone who has dementia will get worse over time and many people will eventually need to be cared for because they cannot live safely alone. It is not uncommon for someone to live seven to ten years after a diagnosis and then to die of something else.

DIAGNOSING AND TREATING DEMENTIA

The prospect of receiving a diagnosis of dementia is frightening. Other conditions such as depression and some physical illnesses (for example, Parkinson's disease) can look like dementia. Dementia can be diagnosed only after careful assessment by a doctor.

In the last 20 years, there has been a great deal of research into treatments of dementia, and drugs are now available to treat memory loss and problems with thinking. There has also been a lot of progress in understanding how someone with dementia, and families and carers, can be supported.

In this book, we describe how dementia is diagnosed and treated. It is important to remember that not all the services and facilities described in this book are available in all areas.

LIVING WITH DEMENTIA

People with dementia can have a good quality of life with help, support and quality care. Dementia is not just about memory loss. Many other problems can occur during the course of the illness, including anxiety, depression, wandering, incontinence and aggression. These can be helped too, and we have included practical advice to help cope with the day-to-day problems that can occur in dementia.

Throughout this book, we have used examples to illustrate some of the problems and difficulties. Although these are based on real patients, we have changed the details to ensure anonymity.

Key points
- The term 'dementia' is used to describe the symptoms that occur when brain function is affected by a variety of different causes. Alzheimer's disease is by far the most common cause
- Dementia is not part of normal ageing
- Dementia is common, affecting over 750,000 people in the UK

2
What Is Dementia?

Mary, a retired factory worker, is 79 and lives alone after her husband died three years ago. Mary is becoming increasingly worried about her memory. Recently she went shopping and left her shopping trolley in the library when she popped in to return a book. On another occasion, she forgot her PIN number when collecting her pension from the post office.

She visited her doctor because she thought she was developing Alzheimer's disease. Dr Thomas listened carefully to her problems and ordered some tests. It turned out Mary did not have dementia. 'As we get older our memory does get worse,' Dr Thomas told her. 'But a problem with memory alone does not mean someone is developing Alzheimer's disease, or any other dementia.'

This chapter explains what dementia is, and outlines the common types of dementia and conditions that can mimic it.

DEFINING DEMENTIA

Dementia is a term that is applied to several different conditions that affect the brain. Just like the word 'arthritis' refers to many different causes of joint pain, there are several different types of dementia, with subtly different symptoms. The most common cause of dementia is Alzheimer's disease, but there are many other causes.

Most kinds of dementia have similar symptoms, including:

- loss of memory, especially for recent events
- problems with thinking and planning
- difficulties with language such as not finding the right words for things
- failure to recognise people or objects
- a change in personality, for example becoming more argumentative
- developing depression, anxiety and other psychological problems.

Our brains (if we think about what our brains do) have many different functions. Making a cup of tea might seem simple but in fact this is quite a complex task and provides examples of several different brain functions:

17

- We imagine a cup of tea (abstract thinking) and decide to make one (motivation).
- We may ask whoever is with us if they want a cup (language).
- We plan making the tea, ensuring that things are done in the right order, putting the tea in before the boiling water (executive function).
- We remember where the tea, sugar and milk are stored (memory).
- We recognise the teapot and kettle (recognition).
- We put the kettle on and gather the ingredients (motor function).
- We listen for the kettle (hearing), ensuring that we don't get distracted with some other task (attention and concentration).
- We carefully pour (coordination) just the right amount of water (judgement) on to the tea.
- We may then add milk and sugar to the cup, in the right order (planning).
- We wait until it has cooled sufficiently (judgement) and we enjoy the tea (taste).
- All the way through we have probably spoken and acted in a similar manner to how we usually do (personality).

Most people reading this book have, at some time or another, made a mistake when making tea. For example, putting tea bags in the fridge and milk in the cupboard instead of the other way round, popping into the next room to ask someone if they want a cuppa and totally forgetting what you wanted to ask or making a cup of tea and forgetting to drink it.

This does not mean that you have dementia. When someone has dementia, usually several of the different brain functions outlined above begin to go wrong, and not just once but repeatedly over time.

So dementia could be defined as: persistent, progressive problems with more than one aspect of brain function (such as language, planning, motivation, memory or personality).

SYMPTOMS OF DEMENTIA

In many types of dementia, problems with memory and complex or abstract thinking are the first symptoms. The memory loss is usually for recent things. So someone may have a clear recollection for things that happened years ago, but cannot remember things that happened a few hours or days ago. People with early dementia sometimes talk a lot about their early life, leading people around them to think their memory is still very good. But when asked about what happened yesterday, the person cannot remember.

Dementia must be differentiated from acute (sudden-onset) causes of confusion. Dementia comes on over months or years; if someone becomes confused over a matter of hours or days this is unlikely to be a dementia.

Acute confusion is usually the result of another physical cause such as:

- infection (for example, chest or urine infection)
- a reaction to medicines
- pain or constipation
- stroke.

Having dementia is a risk factor for getting a more acute confusional state, but, in every case, if someone gets suddenly confused (or more confused), they should see a doctor to try to find the cause of the acute confusion.

People who have dementia can also become more confused if there is a change in routine, such as going on holiday or going into hospital.

Dementia does not always start with memory loss. If an older person develops depression or paranoid thinking that may indicate the start of dementia. Some people with dementia have fairly good memory but may have a change in behaviour, such as irritability or taking risks.

Depression can sometimes mimic dementia.

TYPES OF DEMENTIA

There are over 100 different types and causes of dementia but the great majority of people have one of four types:

1. Alzheimer's disease
2. Vascular dementia

3. Lewy body dementia
4. Frontotemporal dementia.

We shall concentrate on these four. Together, Alzheimer's disease and vascular dementia cause about 90 per cent of all cases of dementia.

Alzheimer's disease

Case study – Gordon

Gordon was 74 when his wife, Liz, first began to notice something was wrong. Looking back, Liz first noticed that Gordon was not looking after his allotment properly. He had been a very keen gardener, often winning prizes for his vegetables. However, Gordon had recently made some mistakes: planting seeds at the wrong time, forgetting to water his plants and letting the weeds get out of control. Neighbours commented that his allotment was a mess.

At first Liz thought Gordon was just bored with gardening, but then other things happened. Gordon was driving back from the supermarket when he suddenly took a wrong turn and went the wrong way up a one-way street.

A few weeks later he got into a muddle with his bank statement and flew into a rage – a very rare thing for him to do.

21

Liz tried to get Gordon to see the doctor but he was adamant that there was nothing wrong. Eventually Liz called Dr Blunt herself, but he told her it was probably just old age and advised her not to worry.

Over the next year things got worse. Gordon began to dress less smartly, sometimes wearing the same clothes until Liz reminded him to change. He began to repeat conversations and would often ask Liz the same question several times over.

He gave up the allotment and would sit for hours doing very little. Liz insisted Gordon went to the doctor and this time she went with him and the doctor took a careful history of Gordon's problems and referred Gordon to the local memory assessment service.

After visiting Gordon and Liz at home and doing some tests, the consultant diagnosed Gordon as having Alzheimer's disease.

Alzheimer's disease is the most common form of dementia; about two-thirds of people with dementia have Alzheimer's disease. This disease was first described over 100 years ago by Alois Alzheimer, who reported on a condition in a woman in her 50s. His description shows the range of symptoms that may develop in this condition:

One of the first disease symptoms of a 51-year-old woman was a strong feeling of jealousy towards her husband. Very soon she showed rapidly increasing memory impairments; she could not find her way about her home, she dragged objects to and fro, hid herself, or sometimes thought that people were out to kill her; then she would start to scream loudly. From time to time she was completely delirious, dragging her blankets and sheets to and fro, calling for her husband and daughter, and seeming to have auditory hallucinations. Often she would scream for hours and hours in a horrible voice. (Alois Alzheimer, 1907)

Alzheimer's disease usually begins with very mild symptoms. The first symptoms are often minor memory loss, which can be difficult to tell from normal forgetfulness as a result of getting older; mild confusion (for example, difficulty managing finances or problems understanding information) and problems with use of language such as not finding the right words may also be present early in the illness. Alzheimer's disease usually starts slowly; it is rare to find someone where the onset can be dated to a particular time, and someone may have the condition for a year or two before it is diagnosed.

Alzheimer's disease also tends to progress slowly. As the disease gets worse, people may have a range of different symptoms and may eventually become very disabled, needing round-the-clock help.

What causes Alzheimer's disease?

Little is known about what triggers the process that leads people to develop Alzheimer's disease. However, scientists now know quite a lot about what happens to the brains of people with Alzheimer's disease. The brain is made up of millions of nerve cells (among other things), which enable us to think and remember.

In a brain affected by Alzheimer's disease, an abnormal protein called amyloid is made (for reasons that are not fully understood). Microscopic amounts of this amyloid protein are laid down in the outer layers of the brain in clumps called plaques (see Figure 2.1).

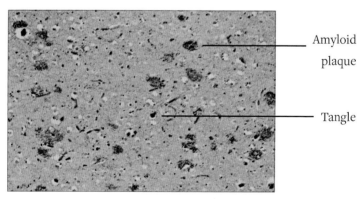

Amyloid plaque

Tangle

Figure 2.1: Picture of microscopic section of brain showing characteristic changes of Alzheimer's disease: tangles and amyloid plaques

These plaques are thought to affect the health of nerve cells or neurons. Neurons contain a protein called tau, which is involved in maintaining the shape of the nerve cell. Affected neurons begin to make an abnormal form of tau, and this is thought to result in a change in the structure of the cells.

Some nerve cells die and collapse in on themselves, creating clumps called tangles. These tangles, and the plaques of amyloid protein, are visible under the microscope and are the hallmarks of Alzheimer's disease.

Certain parts of the brain, especially the temporal lobe (a part of the brain where memory is stored), shrink as a result of the death of neurons. This shrinkage can sometimes be seen on some brain scans and this can help doctors make a diagnosis (Figure 2.2). However, sometimes brain scans can appear normal in people with early Dementia.

The nerve cells in the brain communicate with each other using chemicals called transmitters. In Alzheimer's disease, there are fewer of some of these transmitters, and some treatments for Alzheimer's disease are aimed at increasing the levels of these chemicals (see 'Treatments for Dementia').

Healthy individual   Alzheimer's disease

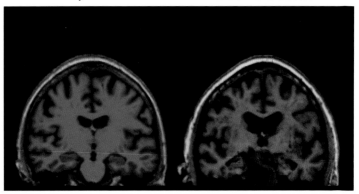

Figure 2.2: Magnetic resonance scan showing a normal
healthy brain and the brain of a person with Alzheimer's
disease on the right, showing thinning of brain tissue

Risk factors for developing Alzheimer's disease

Risk factors are features that increase the chances
that a person will develop dementia. The single most
important risk for developing Alzheimer's disease
is increasing age; as we age beyond 70, the risk for
developing the disease increases considerably.

Other risk factors, such as being female, repeated
head injury (as sustained, for example, by boxers),
high blood pressure, being overweight, diabetes and
smoking, increase the chances of getting Alzheimer's.
Having uncorrected hearing problems may also be a
risk factor.

Drinking small amounts of alcohol (about a glass of
wine) regularly may reduce the risk, but heavy drinking
may increase it.

Factors that may increase the risk of Alzheimer's disease

- Old age
- Genetics (hereditary factors)
- Less education
- High blood pressure
- High cholesterol
- Diabetes
- Obesity
- Deafness
- Social isolation
- Head injury

A family history of Alzheimer's disease

A very small number of people develop Alzheimer's disease in middle age. In these 'young-onset' cases the disease may be caused by an abnormal gene that is passed from one generation to the next. Genes, made up of DNA (deoxyribonucleic acid), are stored in chromosomes, which are found in every cell in the body.

Genes transmit information (for example, characteristics such as skin and eye colour) from one generation to the next. Each person has a pair of genes for each characteristic. Some genes develop abnormalities, called mutations, and these abnormal genes can transmit diseases.

Gene mutations on different chromosomes (chromosomes 1, 14 and 21) have been found that can transmit Alzheimer's disease in this way. If a person has one of these gene mutations they will, on average, pass it to half their children.

Anyone who inherits one of these genes is highly likely to develop Alzheimer's disease, often in their 40s or 50s. However, this is incredibly rare; Alzheimer's disease due to these abnormal genes accounts for less than 1 in every 1000 cases.

If there is a strong family history of Alzheimer's disease starting before the age 60, then doctors may be able to test whether healthy family members are carrying the Alzheimer's disease gene.

The vast majority of people with Alzheimer's disease do not have the type that is passed on from generation to generation by a single gene.

In this 'non-inherited' form of the disease, the risk to close relatives is still higher than for a person of a similar age who has no family history of Alzheimer's disease. For example, someone with no family history has about a 1 in 50 chance of developing Alzheimer's disease during their 70th year. This risk increases to about 1 in 20 in someone with a close relative who did have Alzheimer's disease. The risk is higher still when two close family members are affected. New genes that

may increase the risk of developing Alzheimer's disease

(but do not cause it directly) are being discovered. These may eventually lead to better diagnosis and treatment.

Key features of Alzheimer's disease

- This is the most common cause of dementia
- Over 90 per cent of people with Alzheimers disease are over 70
- It has a slow start with mild symptoms initially
- There is a smooth progression over many years
- Memory is often affected first
- People often live ten years or longer

Vascular dementia

Case study – Pauline

My name is Pauline. I am 69 and worked for many years as a taxi driver. I first noticed something was wrong when I suddenly began to take punters on the wrong route while at work. I was always proud of my 'knowledge' of the streets, so this worried me.

Then one day I felt a bit dizzy and had problems finding the right words to speak. It only lasted 20 minutes or so but I was bothered so went to my GP. By this time my memory was quite bad. My GP organised for me to see a specialist very quickly.

After he did some tests the specialist told me my brain scan showed that I have a poor blood supply to the brain and as a result I have had a lot of mini-strokes ('infarcts' he called them). I didn't realise!

He also tested my memory and said I am in the early stages of vascular dementia. I also have high cholesterol and high blood pressure. I am on aspirin and tablets to control my blood pressure and I have given up smoking.

The second most common cause of dementia is vascular dementia. Around one in five people with dementia has this condition, either on its own or combined with Alzheimer's disease (sometimes called mixed dementia).

Vascular dementia (sometimes known as multi-infarct dementia or vascular cognitive impairment) refers to dementia that occurs because the blood supply to the brain is not as good as it should be or the blood supply to a part of the brain has been interrupted by a stroke or haemorrhage.

The brain needs a great deal of blood to carry oxygen to the nerve cells and receives around a fifth of all the blood that is pumped around the body.

Blood is pumped from the heart through arteries. As these arteries travel deeper into the brain they divide into a multitude of smaller vessels called arterioles. Each arteriole feeds a small section of the brain.

Normally the walls of these arteries and arterioles are smooth, but they may become thickened by fatty deposits called atheroma. This is particularly common in people who smoke or have diabetes or high blood pressure.

When this happens, the artery narrows and the wall becomes roughened. Less blood can get through the narrowed artery, and sometimes the artery wall may develop a clot of blood and block off completely. If this happens in the brain it results in a stroke called an infarct.

Sometimes a short-lived interruption to the blood supply to a region of the brain may not cause any lasting effect. This is known as a transient ischaemic attack (TIA). Symptoms of a TIA last less than 24 hours. A stroke causes lasting damage.

If the blockage resulting in a stroke is in a small artery or arteriole, the resulting stroke may be very small with minor symptoms, but a blockage in a large artery can cause death of a large region of brain and result in death or major symptoms including paralysis, loss of speech or blindness.

Vascular dementia may arise either because the blood supply to the brain is reduced as a result of narrowing of the arteries caused by atheroma, or because of a stroke or series of strokes. Often people have a history of TIAs or several small strokes before they develop vascular dementia, but some people develop vascular dementia with no warning.

Vascular dementia may begin more abruptly than Alzheimer's disease, may deteriorate in steps and may get worse in phases (called step-wise progression) rather than gradually. People with this type of dementia, especially in the early stages, may have lucid intervals (which may be long or short), when they are much more 'with it'.

Symptoms of vascular dementia

The symptoms of vascular dementia can vary depending on which parts of the brain are affected by the poor blood supply. A brain scan can show what areas of the brain are affected.

Often memory and language are affected early, and personality can change early in the disease (for example, people can become more irritable or unmotivated).

People are more likely to be aware of their dementia than if they have Alzheimer's disease. The main finding in the brains of people with vascular dementia is evidence of a reduced flow of blood – often with numerous tiny strokes visible on brain scans.

Key features of vascular dementia

- This is the second most common cause of dementia
- It is caused by a poor blood supply to the brain
- It often starts suddenly and gets worse in steps

Lewy body dementia

Case study – Roy

Roy is 75 and lives alone. He began to have difficulties about three years ago. His first symptom was seeing things that a few seconds later he realised were not there. He often said he saw cats sitting on a chair in his living room but when he looked again they had gone. He also saw a group of children marching up and down silently outside his flat but his neighbour could not see this.

About six months before this, Roy developed a shake on his left hand and had problems walking. His doctor had diagnosed early Parkinson's disease.

When Roy's daughter visited him for a week she got quite worried. She found that Roy was getting up at night and staring at the front door. When she tried to talk to him he seemed unaware that she was there and could not

33

remember anything the following day. She also noticed that Roy seemed quite confused at times, but virtually normal just a few hours later. At his daughter's prompting Roy went to the doctor who diagnosed Lewy body dementia.

Lewy body dementia accounts for about 1 in 20 cases of dementia. It is quite different from Alzheimer's disease and vascular dementia. Early on, people with Lewy body dementia usually have symptoms of Parkinson's disease (shaking, especially in the hands, stiffness and reduced mobility). They also experience hallucinations, often seeing things that are not there (such as people or animals). These hallucinations are often very vivid and detailed but rarely scary.

The difficulties in thinking and memory are similar to Alzheimer's disease but may vary from hour to hour. This variation can be quite dramatic and people can switch quickly – at times people seem fairly normal but can appear confused an hour or so later. People with Lewy body dementia are prone to falls and anxiety. They may have restless nights when they move a lot while dreaming. Sometimes this can get so severe they become quite violent, even though they are asleep. This is called REM (rapid eye movement) sleep disorder.

People who have had Parkinson's disease for many years seem to have a higher risk of developing dementia that is similar to Lewy body dementia. If dementia starts at least a year after the onset of Parkinson's disease it is called Parkinson's disease dementia (PDD).

In common with other types of dementia, older age is a risk factor for developing Lewy body dementia. Other risk factors include being male and having a family history of the disease.

Very little is known about what causes Lewy body dementia. If scientists look at the brains of people with Lewy body dementia they find microscopic lumps of protein in the nerve cells in the brain, called Lewy bodies. These protein deposits disrupt the normal functioning of nerve cells.

Key features of Lewy body dementia

- This is the third most common cause of dementia in UK
- It is more common in men
- People have fluctuating confusion with periods where they may appear normal – at least early on
- People often have vivid visual hallucinations – seeing people or animals
- People have symptoms of Parkinson's disease – shaking and poor mobility

Frontotemporal dementia

Case study – Adam

Adam is 56, divorced and living alone. He was a successful executive in an advertising firm. About four years ago colleagues noticed that Adam was making increasingly outlandish and daring decisions at work.

Some customers liked his 'off-the-wall' suggestions so colleagues didn't worry too much. However, Adam, who had always prided himself on his punctuality, began to miss meetings and turn up late for work. He began to swear and make rude comments to people, both quite uncharacteristic things for him to do.

When Adam began making inappropriate sexual comments to female colleagues, some friends dismissed his behaviour as being caused by the 'male menopause'. One of his friends got really worried and went to see Adam at home and found that he was living in a mess, with stacks of rubbish and boxes of things that he had bought on impulse but never unpacked.

Adam appeared quite unbothered about all this and seemed quite bewildered when the friend expressed concern. Finally, his friends persuaded him to see a doctor. Investigations showed that Adam had a type of dementia called frontotemporal dementia.

About 1 in 50 people with dementia has the frontotemporal type. People with frontotemporal dementia tend to be younger than those with other types of dementia. Of all the types of dementia, frontotemporal dementia is often the most difficult to spot, usually because it affects people in their 50s when dementia is rarely suspected. Although relatively rare overall, frontotemporal dementia affects younger people more and is thought to be as common as Alzheimer's disease in people under 65.

The main area of the brain affected is the frontal lobe, resulting in changes in personality, motivation and increasingly odd or uninhibited behaviour. People affected by this type of dementia may have problems planning and concentrating, and may develop obsessional 'rituals'. Occasionally, people become aggressive or unpredictable. Sometimes people have problems finding the right words, or their speech becomes repetitive or less meaningful.

The areas of the brain mainly involved in memory are affected fairly late in the disease so memory may appear normal at first. The symptoms of frontotemporal dementia are subtle at first and can develop over a very long period of time. Symptoms may be put down to 'midlife crisis' or 'menopause'.

Frontotemporal dementia is usually diagnosed after a brain scan, which may show considerable thinning (atrophy) of the frontal lobe, whereas other parts of the brain may look normal. Cognitive tests can show

37

specific difficulties with tasks dependent on the frontal lobe such as concentration, planning or responding to changing patterns of information.

Some frontotemporal dementia is genetically inherited – about half of all people with it have a family history. It is not known what causes the non-genetic form of the disease.

Dementia related to alcohol

Drinking small amounts of alcohol, say one unit (pub measure) a day, is thought to reduce the risk of developing dementia. However, heavy drinking (several units a day) can increase the chance of dementia.

Case study – Owen

Owen worked as a kitchen fitter. He is divorced and likes a drink. In fact, he was drinking up to ten pints of beer and some scotch a day, every day. One Friday, after fitting a friend's kitchen he left saying he would return on Monday to collect his tools and get paid for the job. Monday came and went but Owen did not show up. The friend could not contact him and got quite worried. Three months passed with no contact then suddenly Owen turned up and asked for his tools and money. His friend paid him and gave him the tools. Five minutes later Owen knocked again asking for his tools and money. When told

he had just got them he denied this and could
not recall the encounter five minutes previously.
Between fitting the kitchen and calling for his
tools three months later, Owen had developed
Korsakoff's syndrome. Although he could not
remember anything that happened only five
minutes previously, he could clearly recall
the memories laid down before he developed
Korsakoff's – the fact he did the job, the
address and the arrangement to collect his tools
and money.

One specific condition related to prolonged
heavy drinking is known as Korsakoff's syndrome.
Korsakoff's syndrome usually has a sudden onset, often
occurring after a period of acute confusion. Individuals
are unable to lay down any new memories following
the onset of this condition, although memories for
events before the disease are often unaffected.

The result is a very disabling amnesia, but without
the other symptoms of dementia (for example,
language and thinking difficulties or personality
change) described in this book. Korsakoff's syndrome
is thought to result from a deficiency of a vitamin
called thiamine. There is damage to a very specific part
of the brain (called the mamillary bodies), although the
rest of the brain may seem unaffected on a scan.

In addition to Korsakoff's syndrome, prolonged heavy use of alcohol probably causes a dementia with symptoms similar to Alzheimer's disease. Some authorities have estimated that up to ten per cent of all cases of dementia are related to alcohol.

RARER TYPES OF DEMENTIA

There are a very large number of rarer causes of dementia, some of which are described below.

Parkinson's disease dementia

This is similar to Lewy body dementia but the dementia comes on many years after the person develops Parkinson's disease. Eventually about one in four people with Parkinson's disease will develop dementia. People tend to have fewer problems with memory, and more apathy and difficulty with planning compared with someone with Alzheimer's disease.

Huntington's disease

This is an inherited disorder that usually begins between the ages of 30 and 50. People with this condition usually develop severe problems with movement and have difficulty controlling their limbs. Anxiety and depression are common. Dementia usually presents with frontal symptoms (problems with planning and thinking, and changes in personality) rather than memory problems.

Creutzfeldt–Jakob disease

There are several subtypes of this very rare disease, which affects about 100 people in the UK each year. Typical (sporadic) Creutzfeldt–Jakob disease (CJD) generally occurs in people who are elderly.

It is caused by a protein called a prion, although the disease can develop many decades after infection. The risk factors for this condition are not fully known, but in a small proportion of cases it seems to run in families. There is rapid development of dementia, often with blindness and severe difficulties with movement. Death usually occurs within a year of developing the condition.

Variant CJD (vCJD) is rarer than CJD and usually occurs in much younger people, typically in their 20s and 30s. This variant may be related to bovine spongiform encephalopathy (BSE or mad cow disease). The vast majority of cases worldwide have occurred in the UK. This is now very rare indeed. People develop depression or anxiety, and problems with sensation and pain before they show signs of dementia.

HIV-related dementia

About two per cent of people with AIDS (acquired immune deficiency syndrome) will eventually develop dementia, often late in the illness. The main features are slowing of mental processes and worsening memory. The incidence has decreased sharply since successful antiretroviral therapy was introduced.

Progressive supranuclear palsy

In this condition, the nerves controlling balance and movement are damaged, leading to loss of coordination, slurred speech, swallowing difficulties and falls. There may also be personality change. Dementia often occurs after these other symptoms have developed.

CONDITIONS THAT LOOK LIKE DEMENTIA

Case study – Anne

Anne is 74. Her husband died last year and after that Anne began to get more and more forgetful. She had to stop playing cards in the local bridge club because she could not concentrate on the game. Then she forgot that she was due to organise the teas at a local Women's Institute (WI) meeting – a very embarrassing mistake for her.

Things then went from bad to worse. She lost her energy and found even simple things, like hanging out the washing, difficult to do. Eventually she spent more and more time just sitting at home doing nothing. She could not remember the plot of the book she was reading and lost interest in the TV.

When her doctor suggested that Anne may be depressed she didn't agree; she didn't feel sad or tearful. She was worried that she had

Alzheimer's disease, having seen a friend develop it a couple of years earlier.

However, after a course of treatment for depression her energy levels and concentration returned and her memory began to improve. Three months on she is back playing bridge and doing the teas at the WI.

There are many conditions that cause slowly progressive memory loss and confusion that look like dementia. Some of these are treatable. This is one reason why it is so important for people who have symptoms such as memory loss or change in personality to see a doctor for a full check-up.

Depression

Depression will affect one in three people at some point in their lives. In older people in particular it can be mistaken for dementia because many of the symptoms are the same.

People with depression may complain of feeling low or depressed, may lack energy or lose a sense of enjoyment. Often nothing can brighten them up. It is common for people with depression to think about suicide. Untreated, these feelings will last for months.

Other symptoms include poor sleep (especially waking early), loss of appetite, and poor concentration and memory. These are also common symptoms of dementia. An added complication is that people with dementia are even more likely to get depression as well – as many as half the people with dementia will get depressed.

Things that may point to depression rather than dementia include:

- feeling worse in the morning (as a rule people with dementia tend to be brighter in the mornings)
- having thoughts of guilt, worthlessness or suicide
- low mood, which is sustained over weeks.

Depression is under-recognised and is a miserable state to be in. With treatment, depression can get completely better. If you or someone you know may have depression, it is important to seek medical help quickly.

Underactive thyroid gland
Also called hypothyroidism, this can start gradually and be difficult to spot. People with this condition may feel cold all the time, their skin may get coarse and dry, and they generally feel tired and 'slowed up'. A blood test will confirm the diagnosis.

Parkinson's disease
This is quite a common disorder in older people.

People with Parkinson's disease may notice shaking or tremor (which often starts in one hand), which is more noticeable when relaxing, and stiffness in their arms and legs. People with Parkinson's disease show less facial expression and may have problems walking. Although some people with Parkinson's disease develop dementia, others don't but being slowed up in thinking and speaking may make it seem as if the person has dementia.

Delirium/acute confusional state

Case study – Eve

Eve was fine when she went into hospital for her hip replacement. The operation went well but three days later Eve suddenly became confused one evening. She started shouting at her husband that she had been moved to a different hospital and the nurses were not real nurses. She would not eat her dinner because she was convinced it was poisoned. When the doctor saw her she did not know what the time or date was. The following morning she was a little better but became confused and agitated again later in the day. The doctor did some tests and found that Eve had a chest infection. After a few days of antibiotics and oxygen, Eve was much more settled and less confused.

Sometimes people can get confused over a matter of hours or days. This is not dementia but something that doctors call delirium, or acute confusional state.

One of the main differences from dementia is that delirium starts very quickly. Also, people with delirium may be drowsy or become suddenly agitated. They often have difficulty focusing on a topic and are inattentive.

People who have delirium often change rapidly; for example, they may appear quite calm one minute and become very distressed, agitated or aggressive the next. They often hallucinate (see things that are not there). Behaviour is usually more disturbed at night.

Many things can cause delirium, commonly chest or urine infections, heart failure, prescribed medicines, alcohol or a stroke. If someone develops an acute confusion they should see a doctor or be taken to the hospital urgently.

Conditions that can mimic dementia
- Depression
- Underactive thyroid gland
- Acute confusion (delirium)
- Some vitamin deficiencies (e.g. vitamin B12)
- Some infections
- Rarely, a brain tumour can look like dementia

Key points

- Dementia is a disease; it is not caused by normal ageing
- The most common type of dementia is Alzheimer's disease, although there are many other causes
- Many conditions look like dementia; anyone who develops symptoms of confusion should see a doctor

3
Symptoms of Dementia

HOW DEMENTIA STARTS

Dementia often begins subtly; when people with dementia and their families look back on when the first symptoms started, it is often difficult to date.

Sometimes people first notice a problem when the person with dementia has their routine changed; for example, when they go on holiday or become ill. The death of a partner can sometimes reveal dementia in the surviving partner. Bereavement does not cause dementia but may reveal it because the person who has died had been helping out.

In the UK, the proportion of people with dementia who get a diagnosis has increased in recent years. A few years ago, only one in three ever received a diagnosis, now it is closer to two in three. This still means a third of people with dementia never get diagnosed. Of those who do, it often takes one to two years between the start of symptoms and someone seeing a doctor.

The earlier the diagnosis is made the better. If you

suspect that you, or someone close to you, are developing dementia, seek medical advice sooner rather than later.

An accurate diagnosis of dementia rules out the possibility of a different treatable condition such as depression that may look like dementia. It provides the person, and their family with an explanation for the new symptoms.

It also allows people with dementia and their carers to better plan and prepare for the future, for example by setting up a lasting power of attorney and planning their care. It also allows earlier access to treatment and management advice.

THE PROGRESSION OF DEMENTIA

Dementia is usually a progressive disease. It affects people in different ways. This is because the symptoms and the way in which they develop reflect personality, lifestyle, quality of relationships, and mental and physical health.

Symptoms vary with the different types of dementia but there are some broad similarities between them all. Most common are loss of memory and loss of practical abilities, leading to a loss of independence and affecting social relationships.

The course of the disease is very variable. People may live with disease for over 20 years but it could be much less than this. In the end, people with dementia usually die of some other condition, such as a heart attack or an infection, which may be quite unconnected to the dementia.

Over recent years, better care and understanding have generally led to a greater expectation of life, and quality of life, for people with dementia. It is important to come to terms with dying with dementia and to make plans for death. If you have dementia it is helpful to discuss what treatments you would or would not want to have when you reach the final stages.

Although dementia progresses at different rates in different people, it is helpful to describe the progress of the disease at an early stage, as the disease progresses, and at the late stage. This is a rough guide only. No one will have all the symptoms listed but this summary can help people with dementia and their carers to understand what they are likely to expect and help them to plan for the future.

Early stage

Case study – Bev

When Bev and Richard looked back, there were several clues over the years. Her love of gardening faded; sometimes she just seemed a bit vague; she stopped doing the crossword puzzle. The very first thing that they noticed was that Bev was less able to hold conversations on the phone. She was okay if she was making the call, but got quite confused if someone else rang her.

The onset of dementia is usually very gradual so that it is difficult to know when it actually starts. This stage is often overlooked and it is only when people are helped to look back in time that they realise that odd symptoms did occur but their significance was not recognised or they were excused as being part of normal ageing.

A person in the early stage may:

- become forgetful, especially of things that have just happened
- lose their sense of time, leading to missing appointments or not paying bills
- show loss of interest and poor concentration
- lose motivation
- become more withdrawn
- have language problems, with difficulty finding the right words
- show odd behaviour
- have difficulty making decisions
- be less engaged with family/company
- be 'different' from their old self
- show mood changes and be depressed or easily irritable.

Middle stage

This is a time when it is clear that a person has dementia and that it is affecting everyday functioning and the ability to live independently. This can give rise to changes in behaviour often through frustration and a lack of understanding on the part of the person with the dementia and the carer.

The person with dementia at this stage may:

- become more forgetful – they might forget names of family and close friends and recent events, which can often give rise to repetitive questioning
- walk out of the house and get lost
- not be able to work out the difference between day and night and have difficulty sleeping
- have difficulties understanding what is being said
- have increased difficulty with speech
- have problems with household tasks such as cleaning and cooking
- need help with dressing and washing and need reminding to go to the toilet
- lose things and blame others for taking them
- become aggressive
- experience hallucinations.

Late stage

This is when the person with dementia has very serious memory problems and becomes completely dependent on others for their physical care. They may:

- have great difficulty communicating
- have poor or no recognition of family and friends

- not understand what is said to them or what is going on around them
- need help with eating
- be incontinent of urine and faeces
- have difficulty walking
- have difficulty swallowing
- be chair and bed bound.

This stage can last months or years, depending on the physical health of the person and the quality of the care that the person is receiving. Death may be caused by infections, strokes or heart attacks.

Final stage

Case study – Peter

Peter had Alzheimer's disease for 12 years. In the last year he was in a nursing home unable to care for himself. He needed help with everything, including eating and washing, and could not get out of bed. He had been nursed in bed for six months and in that time had not spoken a word. He seemed oblivious to his surroundings, not communicating or seeming to take any interest in what was going on around him. Eventually he developed pneumonia and the nurses thought he would die that night. They consulted his end-of-life care plan, which Peter had written with his wife and GP some years earlier, after

53

his diagnosis. This stated that Peter did not want to die in hospital. So the nurses made him comfortable in the nursing home and called his wife to let her know. His wife Helen visited that evening. Peter was close to death. He opened his eyes, stretched out his hand and touched her arm and said, 'Hello darling, I love you.' Six hours later Peter passed away peacefully.

By this stage, the person will be unable to speak or move properly; they will need full care, including help with eating and drinking.

Often in the last stages swallowing becomes difficult. It is important to understand that even in the final stages of dementia people will often be aware of their surroundings, who is around them, and what is being said, as is shown in Peter's story. Almost certainly they will be able to feel pain (for example, from toothache or constipation) and will feel uncomfortable if hungry or dehydrated.

DIAGNOSIS OF DEMENTIA

Recognising the symptoms of dementia is the first step towards receiving a diagnosis and getting help. If you or your relative are worried that you are depressed or forgetful or showing any of the signs described above then going to your GP is the first thing to do.

Early and accurate diagnosis is helpful for several reasons:

- It provides an explanation for symptoms and changes in behaviour and helps the people with dementia and their carers to be better equipped to deal with the disease and know what to expect as time goes on.
- It allows people to understand what is happening to them and to have some control over their life. For example, they can decide on treatments and future care, write wills, take a holiday, see distant relatives, and set up financial and welfare powers of attorney.
- Appropriate support services and financial help can be put in place and help people to plan for the future.
- It can ensure that other problems that can lead to memory loss, such as depression, are dealt with appropriately.
- For a number of people with dementia – and it is not possible yet to predict which ones – medication offers the possibility of slowing the disease process. Obviously, if the diagnosis is not made for whatever reason, it is not possible to offer such treatment.

How the diagnosis is made

There is no simple test to make the diagnosis of dementia. A diagnosis is made by taking a careful account from the person with the problem and, even more importantly, from a close relative or friend.

Seeing the doctor

The first step to getting a diagnosis is to see a doctor. It takes some courage to suggest to someone close to you that they may need help. And it takes courage for the person with dementia to take the first step. There is still a lot of worry and stigma about getting a diagnosis of dementia, which puts some people off. However, most people who take the first step to getting a diagnosis are pleased they did.

It can be quite difficult to get help if someone resolutely refuses to do anything. If someone refuses to see a doctor at all, then consider speaking directly with their GP or social services on that person's behalf. If you are worried about someone, it is worth persevering to get help because without it, life with dementia can be risky and miserable. You could try to get the person you are worried about to the doctor for an 'annual health check'. Ultimately the GP may call a specialist to visit the person at home.

Often people with dementia are not aware of all their difficulties, so it may be necessary for someone to accompany them to the doctor when they do go. The GP will want to ask some questions about memory and difficulties with day-to-day tasks and will probably do a short memory test. They may organise some tests themselves or they may refer on to a local specialist.

Specalist referral

In the last few years, memory services have been set up in many parts of the UK. If the GP thinks someone may have dementia they will probably refer to the local memory service in the first instance, or to the local hospital. During the assessment, you may see:

- an old age psychiatrist (a doctor specialising in the mental disorders of old age)
- a neurologist (a specialist in diseases of the nervous system)
- a geriatrician (a specialist in medical diseases of older people).

Exactly which specialist someone is referred to will depend on their age, what symptoms they have and what services are available locally. Sometimes it may be necessary for a person to see more than one specialist; for example, a neurologist may ask an old age psychiatrist for a second opinion if symptoms of depression are present.

The specialist may see the person in a memory service or hospital outpatients or go to see the person at home. Old age psychiatrists, in particular, often see a patient at home in the first instance. Seeing someone at home is not only usually more convenient for the patient but also allows the doctor to assess the home environment and gauge how well someone is coping at home.

Although the doctor will almost certainly want to ask someone else (usually a close relative or friend) for their account, they may want to speak to the person alone to begin with.

When seeing a doctor, it is helpful to go prepared with some notes of the concerns that you have, the symptoms that you have noticed and when they started to occur. Often the assessment may take place on a single day, or may be done over a few weeks.

The doctor will normally ask questions about:

- the symptoms, especially when they were first noticed and how they have progressed and developed
- how the symptoms affect life and day-to-day tasks
- the person's past history, including medical history and medication
- the person's previous personality
- family history
- the person's views about the symptoms.

The doctor should build up an account of the person, known as a life story, so that they can see the difficulties in the context of the individual.

The assessment should include a physical examination to check that the heart and lungs are working properly, to check for signs of neurological illness such as Parkinson's disease or stroke, and to assess the risk of falls.

A psychological assessment should check for symptoms of depression, anxiety and psychosis (for example, having hallucinations).

Memory and cognitive tests

It is common practice to carry out a simple test of memory and thinking. There are numerous tests but one most commonly used is the Montreal Cognitive Assessment (MOCA). The test takes about ten minutes. The doctor asks a series of questions including remembering some words to be recalled later, drawing a clock, copying a diagram, recognising some pictures of animals, repeating some phrases and numbers and the date, and saying where the person is now.

The MOCA has a top score of 30. People with dementia often score below 26, but some people with higher scores can still have dementia. As dementia progresses, the MOCA score will drop. Scores below ten indicate quite severe dementia.

For some people the doctor may refer for a more in-depth test of memory and thinking (called neuropsychometry), which is usually done by a psychologist (a specialist in mental processes such as memory). These tests can take up to two hours, give a detailed profile of changes in brain function and help map which parts of the brain (for example, the frontal lobe) are most affected in an individual. This can also estimate whether there has been a decrease compared with what would be expected for that individual.

Occupational therapist

Another person involved in the assessment could be an occupational therapist, who may conduct an assessment at home or in a special area in the hospital. This can be helpful in assessing skills with activities of daily living and areas where a person may need help or adaptations. It can also assess the environment and identify what changes or equipment may help maintain independence and reduce risks.

The assessment should check whether there are risks (for example, tripping on stairs or getting lost) and whether the person is getting enough food and can prepare meals. Looking in the fridge of someone who has dementia can reveal a great deal!

Social worker

A social worker may be involved in the assessment. Social workers can assess what practical help a person needs and arrange for this to be supplied. People with dementia are at risk of financial exploitation; finances may need safeguarding, through either appointeeship or the Court of Protection – something else that a social worker can help with.

Other investigations

Many people suspected of having dementia will have other investigations that are usually arranged by the specialist. These may include:

- CT brain scan (computed tomography)
- MRI (magnetic resonance imaging)
- Amyloid PET scan (positron emission tomography).

These scans provide detailed images of the brain and can show areas of shrinkage or damage such as that caused by a stroke. All the scans involve lying on a small trolley and being moved into the scanner.

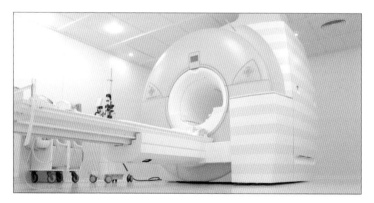

Figure 3.1: An MRI scanner

MRI uses a strong magnetic pulse to visualise the structure of the brain and can produce very detailed images. An MRI scan can take about half an hour;

61

it is important to lie still and it can feel quite claustrophobic and noisy (see Figure 3.1).

A CT scan uses a small dose of X-rays to create pictures of the brain. Although it is not as detailed as an MRI scan, the image can still be useful. It takes only a few minutes to do a CT scan.

An amyloid PET scan uses a chemical with a small amount of radioactivity which binds to amyloid, the protein laid down in the brains of people with Alzheimer's disease. Where amyloid is present the brain lights up on the scan pictures. PET scans are less common than MRI and CT scans but may be used where the diagnosis is not clear (see Figure 3.2).

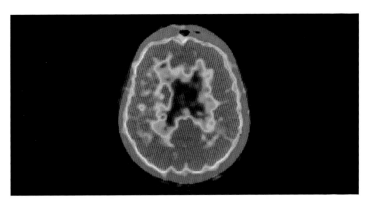

Figure 3.2: A PET scan image

The results of these scans can take some weeks to get back. Almost certainly the doctor will order some blood tests to check for anaemia, inflammation, vitamin levels, the health of the thyroid gland, and kidney and liver function. These results are normally back in a few days.

Other tests may include a brain-wave trace (electroencephalogram or EEG) and lumbar puncture. EEG involves wearing something like a swimming cap with lots of wires coming off it. These traces can sometimes help distinguish different types of dementia but are not done often. A lumbar puncture involves drawing a small amount of fluid off the spine for analysis of amyloid, but is very rarely recommended.

Discussing the diagnosis

When the tests are finished, the doctor should sit down and be prepared to discuss the diagnosis with the person. It may be helpful to have a friend or family member there. Most people with dementia want to know the diagnosis, whereas many family members prefer that their relative is not told. Being open about the diagnosis of dementia is important.

The doctor should ask whether the person wants to hear the diagnosis and, if they do, should explain this clearly and simply. This is a good opportunity also to discuss treatments, what help may be needed, and what practical, emotional and financial support is available. It is also helpful to discuss plans for the future, such as writing advance directives.

It will normally take some time to come to terms with the diagnosis. Over time you should try to ensure you have discussed the following points:

- What type of dementia is it?
- What treatments are available?
- What benefits can I get?
- What other help and support is available to me?
- How is it likely to progress?
- Can I set up lasting powers of attorney for finance and for health?
- Can I write a will?
- What is end-of-life care planning?
- What about my driving?

It is usually difficult to take everything in at one go so a follow-up appointment with a counsellor or the doctor can be helpful.

Key points
- Getting a diagnosis is the first step to getting help and support
- Everyone with dementia should be offered the chance to hear the diagnosis
- The assessment should include checking physical, psychological and social factors
- Support and advice after diagnosis are very important

4
Treatments for Dementia

CAN DEMENTIA BE TREATED?

It is important to emphasise that the mainstay of dementia care is not about drug treatment. Providing practical and emotional support, advocacy and information to the individual with dementia and their carers and family is a huge part of dementia treatment.

It is often thought that dementia cannot be treated. It is true that it cannot be cured, but there is a great deal that can be done to help. This is the focus of this chapter and the next.

Case study – Joyce

My name is Joyce and I have been getting more forgetful for three years. At first, I put this down to getting old but, when I began to lose the thread of conversations and got lost returning from the local shops, I talked to my husband Eric and we decided to get help. I went with my husband to our GP who referred me to the local hospital.

After tests confirmed I probably had Alzheimer's disease, the consultant started me on an anti-dementia drug. After three months on the medicine, I felt more confident in talking to my husband and able to go to the shops on my own again.

This chapter explains the treatments that are available for dementia, including treatments for memory and challenging behaviour.

PREVENTING DEMENTIA

There are some things we cannot change that increase our risk of getting dementia. These include getting older, our family history and our level of education. However, some lifestyle characteristics also appear to be associated with an increased risk of getting dementia. Correctable lifestyle factors which appear to increase risk of dementia include:

- hearing loss
- physical inactivity
- high blood pressure
- diabetes
- obesity
- smoking

- social isolation
- drinking excess alcohol.

Except for getting older and having a strong family history, none of these risk factors has a strong link with dementia and scientists often disagree on what risks are important. However, in the last few years the incidence (number of new cases in a defined population) of dementia has fallen, possibly because of the improved health of the population, so a healthy lifestyle may well be very important to prevent dementia in some people.

Some scientists have suggested that taking aspirin, antioxidants such as vitamin E or cholesterol-lowering drugs called statins may reduce the chance of getting dementia, but this needs further investigation.

It also seems that people who keep their brains active may be at less risk of developing dementia. Reading, engaging in a hobby such as playing bridge or chess, or doing crosswords and word puzzles may help reduce the risk.

Perhaps the best advice is to:

- get your hearing checked
- exercise your body regularly
- exercise your brain regularly
- meet other people
- keep to a healthy diet
- drink alcohol sensibly

- don't smoke
- have regular check-ups to exclude diabetes and high blood pressure.

TREATING DEMENTIA

There are two sets of symptoms that may need treatment in dementia. The first is the treatment of cognitive symptoms (memory loss, problems with thinking and confusion).

The second is the treatment of behavioural and psychological symptoms of dementia, such as depression, anxiety, hallucinations, and irritable or aggressive behaviour, which tend to occur later in the condition.

There are frequent and often wildly exaggerated claims for new treatments in the press; these raise expectations but rarely fulfil their promise.

Treatment of memory loss and other cognitive symptoms

Case study – Ben

Ben is a keen gardener. When the doctor visited him at home he was happy to show off his garden. However, he became frustrated when he could not recall the names of the plants. Three months after starting donepezil, the doctor visited again and, to her delight, Ben could recall the names of most of the plants.

Medication

Until about 20 years ago there were virtually no useful drug treatments for cognitive symptoms of dementia. Now, the mainstay of treatment of memory loss in Alzheimer's disease is a group of drugs known as cholinesterase inhibitors.

There are currently three drugs in this category:

1. Donepezil (Aricept)
2. Galantamine (Reminyl)
3. Rivastigmine (Exelon).

They all work by increasing the levels of a chemical transmitter in the brain called acetylcholine (ACh). The theory is that, by boosting this chemical, nerve cells involved in memory should be able to communicate better with each other.

Some people have a definite improvement in their memory and thinking after taking these drugs, although others seem to have no benefit. Unfortunately, it is not possible to predict who will and who will not benefit; the only way to tell is to try the drugs.

These medicines need to be taken every day for some weeks before an effect is likely to be seen. If one doesn't work there is probably little point in trying another. However, some people who get side effects with one drug may cope better with one of the other drugs.

These medicines usually need to be started by a specialist. The doctor will probably want to check some things, including a heart trace (electrocardiogram or ECG), before starting any of these drugs.

These drugs have some side effects, although many people find them quite easy to take and don't have any side effects. The main side effects that people may experience are feeling sick (nausea), diarrhoea and stomach pains. For many people, these side effects improve in a few days.

The current anti-dementia drugs do not stop the disease from progressing. For someone who is responding to treatment it may make the difference between, say, being able and not being able to cook meals or remember to pay bills. In other words, some people may be able to stay independent for longer.

Once the person has taken the tablets for between three and six months the doctor should check whether they are helping. Between one in three and one in four people who take these medicines has a definite improvement and would benefit from staying on them.

Deciding whether the medicine is helping can be difficult; probably the best marker of response is the view from the patient and family/friends about whether there has been any improvement or deterioration. Doctors may use a cognitive test such as the Montreal Cognitive Examination (MOCA) to help decide whether someone is responding to anti-dementia medicines. After six months, someone with untreated dementia should normally show a lower (worse) score. If the score is unchanged, or better than when the medicines were started, this would indicate that the medicine may be working.

Cognitive stimulation therapy

This is a talking treatment where people either individually or in groups, once or twice a week, do a variety of activities such as quizzes or word games, discussing current affairs or talking about their childhood. It is thought the social aspect of the activity and the activity itself are both helpful in improving memory. Research has suggested cognitive stimulation therapy does help many people with dementia and may be as effective as tablets.

Memantine

A drug that acts on another memory chemical in the brain called NMDA (N-methyl-d-aspartate) has been used for the treatment of later stages of dementia and may improve behaviours such as irritability and agitation.

Ginkgo biloba

Ginkgo biloba is a natural extract from the maidenhair tree and is promoted as a treatment to help memory. Clinical trials in dementia show variable results and Ginkgo may not be an effective treatment.

Aspirin

Aspirin and other non-steroidal, anti-inflammatory drugs have been suggested, but there is insufficient research to be certain whether these are helpful.

Many other treatments have been investigated but none has been shown to be effective.

Treatment of behavioural symptoms

Case study – Richard

Richard lived with his partner, Andrew, in a basement flat. Richard had developed dementia about four years ago and was becoming a bit of a handful. He was incontinent of urine and most afternoons got quite agitated, trying to get out of the flat and shouting that he wanted to go home. He did not recognise that the flat was his home!

Andrew was very keen to care for Richard at home, but was finding it increasingly difficult. The local hospital sent a community nurse who specialised in dementia. She gave Andrew advice about how to deal with Richard's incontinence, including taking him to the toilet regularly and using special pads.

The nurse also suggested that, instead of trying to keep Richard in the flat in the afternoon, as soon as he became agitated, Andrew should take him for a walk around the block. When he did this, Richard was much more settled in the evenings.

When Alois Alzheimer first described Alzheimer's disease, he noted that some of the most difficult symptoms were not to do with memory but changes in mood and behaviour. Nearly all people with dementia will experience some changes in behaviour or mood and many will experience multiple symptoms. Many of these symptoms can cause a great deal of distress for people with dementia and those caring for them. Some, such as depression, can make the memory problems worse and may reduce the ability to do everyday tasks.

TABLE 4.1: CHANGES IN BEHAVIOUR AND EMOTION IN DEMENTIA

Very common	Common	Less common
Apathy	Verbal or physical aggression	Crying
Restlessness		Repetitive actions
Eating problems	Agitation	Hallucinations
Sleeping problems	Screaming	
Depression	Sexual problems	
Anxiety	Paranoid thinking	
Repeated questioning		

Sometimes a physical reason, such as a urine infection or constipation, is the cause of the symptoms. For these reasons, anyone showing any of these symptoms should be seen by a doctor to exclude a physical cause. Once a physical cause has been ruled out, the treatment depends on the symptom.

It is helpful to see these symptoms in the context

of the person, and the past and current environment. To enable this a 'life story' can be extremely helpful. A life story builds up a profile of the person: their background, education, hobbies, career, relationships and personality characteristics.

Building a life story with the help of the person with dementia and their family and friends can be very useful if someone enters a care home, as the staff caring for the person will have a far better understanding of the person. This can take the form of an album, with photographs.

In recent years, there has been a huge shift away from using medicines to control behaviour problems in people with dementia. Only after looking for physical causes, such as infections and pain, and making sure the person has sufficient exercise, human contact and has adequate and appropriate activities should drugs be considered. It is no longer appropriate to just diagnose 'behavioural problems' and give a catch-all sedative. It is recognised there are several subtypes of behavioural and psychological symptoms of dementia and these should be individually addressed.

Whatever the cause of dementia, the behavioural and psychological symptoms are likely to change in type and severity as the illness progresses. For this reason, people should have their treatment reviewed regularly.

Depression

Case study – Alice

Music was Alice's first and greatest love. She had been in various choirs since the age of eight. She was an accomplished pianist and also played the flute. She worked as a volunteer for many years, teaching music in the local prison. She had a huge collection of classical music records.

Alice had Alzheimer's disease for eight years and had recently moved into a residential home. Although she visited the home before moving in, and seemed to like it, once there she became increasingly anxious, depressed and irritable.

She would pace around the corridors and sometimes shout out if she was sat in front of the television. The staff in the home were aware of Alice's life story and thought that she was upset because she had been deprived of her music. Her grandson came to the rescue; he bought an MP3 player and put a lot of her music onto it. Alice now listens to her music frequently and seems more content.

Depression is difficult to diagnose in dementia. People often lack the ability to say they are feeling sad. Depression can make many symptoms of dementia, such as forgetfulness, poor concentration and lack of motivation, even worse. If someone with dementia is suspected of having depression they should be seen by a doctor urgently because they may need antidepressants (tablets that help depression).

Crying

Crying can occur even if someone does not seem depressed. Sometimes people just go from being happy to crying and back to happy, like flicking a switch. This is called emotional lability. It is often upsetting for onlookers but the person with lability may not appear distressed. Sometimes antidepressants can help.

Agitation and restlessness

Repetitive, purposeless movements and pacing around may be the result of pain or discomfort or a sign of boredom, but often just happen with no explanation. These are some of the most distressing symptoms for the carer but sometimes do not appear to be distressing for the person with dementia.

If it is not too extreme, the best thing may be just to tolerate the restlessness. However, sometimes adjusting the routine may help to reduce the problem.

The mainstay of treatment is analysing the behaviour to find out the causes and consequences, which may help to find the solution, as shown in the next case.

Case study – James

James was a big man – well over six feet tall. He cut quite a striking figure in the nursing home where he lived. James had vascular dementia, which affected his speech, and one of his major problems was that he found it very difficult to make himself understood.

Over some weeks James became more aggressive, sometimes hitting staff or other residents. The staff at the home were at the end of their tether and demanded that James be moved to a hospital.

An analysis of this behaviour showed that most of James's aggression took place around meal times. The nurse observed that when the food was being served James became increasingly agitated and sometimes aggressive, and that the longer James had to wait for his food the worse things became.

Also, it seemed as if James was still hungry after the meal (he was receiving the same size portions as all the other residents). They decided to try giving James his food first and to give him an extra helping; this worked like a dream. The aggression subsided and James was able to continue living in the home.

In the past, these problems were often treated using antipsychotic drugs such as haloperidol or risperidone, but these drugs have been found to be harmful in some people with dementia (they may cause falls, excessive sedation, stroke and early death) and should be used only in the most extreme situations when prescribed by a specialist.

Some non-antipsychotic drugs may help agitation and restlessness. These include memantine, which has been shown to help agitation in some people, and trazodone, which can help restlessness at night.

In Lewy body dementia, people with night-time agitation (REM sleep disorder) respond well to a medicine called clonazepam.

Eating problems

People with dementia experience changes in taste for food and appetite. They may find it hard to tell people they are hungry. Many people lose weight once they develop dementia, despite getting more of a taste for sweet foods. A more flexible approach to meals – possibly serving finger food or smaller meals more often, and changing the diet to suit the individual – can help.

Sleeping problems

Not being able to sleep at night is a common difficulty. People may get up in the early hours and think it is daytime; they may get dressed and try to go to work.

Sleep problems at night are often made worse by napping during the day and lack of exercise.

The first step should be getting into a routine with exercise and fresh air every day, not having 'cat naps', and avoiding heavy meals or stimulating drinks (such as coffee) before bedtime. Thick curtains may help stop someone waking early, and a clock by the bed may help remind them it's night-time. If nothing helps, doctors may prescribe a sedative, but these can cause falls and worse confusion so need to be used cautiously.

Disinhibition

Disinhibition is the loss of usual control over our impulses. For example, if we see a very attractive person we may have the desire to kiss them, but usually we would stop ourselves from doing this.

Disinhibition can be one of the most difficult symptoms to cope with. People may say cutting or hurtful things or behave inappropriately – for example, urinating in public, or making sexual suggestions to family, friends or passers-by. These can be difficult to treat and may require a specialist opinion. Sometimes, in extreme cases, sedatives may be needed to reduce the behaviour.

Sexual problems

Sexual problems, such as excessive demands for sex, masturbating in public, touching the genitalia or making sexual demands on strangers, can be very embarrassing and upsetting for partners and carers.

It has to be remembered at all times that this behaviour is due to the disease not the person. It can be equally upsetting if a person no longer wants to have sex and the partner feels very rejected. If any of these problems occur, it can be helpful to talk things over with a specialist nurse or doctor who can often make helpful suggestions. Sometimes drugs can be used to reduce sex drive.

Equally frustrating (for a partner) can be a loss of sex drive that may accompany dementia. Libido will vary over time, but persistent loss of sexual relations can happen. Trying different ways to rekindle a partner's interest in sex may help.

Delusions and hallucinations

Delusions (the person believing that someone is stealing things or trying to harm them) and hallucinations (seeing or hearing things that are not there) are often seen in people with dementia.

If these are not causing distress, it may be best to leave them alone. A group of drugs called antipsychotics may help reduce these symptoms but there are risks and these should be prescribed only by a specialist who reviews the person regularly.

Key points

- Keeping your body healthy and brain active may help to prevent dementia
- Memory loss and other cognitive symptoms may be helped by treatment with anti-dementia drugs called cholinesterase inhibitors
- Behavioural symptoms should be seen in the context of the life story – sedative drugs should be given only as a last resort

5
Getting Help

HOW TO GET HELP – WHO PAYS?

Help is available from a variety of sources and all the professionals discussed in this chapter may be useful. Any person with dementia and their carer are entitled to a needs assessment, which is normally carried out by an appropriately trained assessor, such as a social worker or an occupational therapist from the local social services department.

Under the Care Act 2014 you have a right to be assessed for free by your local council if you appear to need care and support to complete activities in your day-to-day life. You have this right to be assessed regardless of your financial situation. This assessment is free but you may have to ask for it. You can ring the local social services department, or your GP may be able to put you in touch. The assessment may reveal a number of needs for which help is required. After this process of assessment is finished, the decision can then be made about whether you are entitled to care and support arranged by the local authority.

A named key worker, usually the social worker, will draw up a care plan to promote your independence and well-being and discuss your needs and work with you to find out what is available locally. The sort of help available may include information, care at your home, such as help with shopping and cleaning, meals on wheels, adult day care centres and respite. This help is usually means-tested so you may have to pay for it yourself or make a contribution to the cost. It is up to your local council to decide if and how much to charge, but they have limits. At the moment, your capital and savings below £14,250 are disregarded in the means test.

If you have:

- between £14,250 and £23,250 in capital and savings and you are eligible for care, the council will contribute towards your care costs
- capital and savings above £23,250, you will have to fund all of your own social care.

When your care and support needs are assessed by the council, you will also be asked to complete a financial assessment. This means assessment will determine if, and how much, you should pay towards your care and support services. The assessment will only look at your individual means, not the means of any other family member, even if they are looking after your financial affairs on your behalf.

The Care Act 2014 stated that from April 2015 councils had to assign a personal budget to all people eligible for support, and local authorities are increasingly using this process. The personal budget is an allocation of funding paid to someone so that they can arrange for the help that they need themselves (with the help of their family if necessary). Personal budgets give the person more flexibility and control, but arranging and supervising care can be stressful. If you are eligible for a personal budget, you can ask your council to spend your personal budget and organise your support for you. Or you can ask them to give your personal budget money to you in the form of a direct payment followed by a care and support plan showing how the personal budget will be used to meet your assessed needs. You can form the plan yourself, with family and friends, or with help from social services or another organisation. If you choose to have a direct payment, you will need to sign both the plan and a direct payment agreement – a contract with the council – outlining your responsibilities.

TYPES OF HELP

All people with dementia and their carers will need help. The types of assistance most frequently needed are:

- information
- practical help
- medical help
- personal support.

Support and services for people with dementia vary widely around the country – in some areas they may be very good, in others they may be limited. It is hoped that the National Dementia Strategy in England, and similar developments in other countries, will ensure that good services are more widely available.

Information

Information is going to be needed on all aspects of dementia, and on where to find help. Most information can be obtained free (online, library, GP surgery, Citizens Advice service or local council) but you might want to buy one or two books. The information required will change as time goes on. Some financial benefits are available for people with dementia and their carers, and advice and information on these, together with advice on arranging a will or a lasting power of attorney, will be required. Some people living with dementia, and their carers, may have financial worries and they should ask a professional, such as a social worker, about different types of benefits that may be available to them. You may want to ask about Attendance Allowance, Carer's Allowance, Carer's Credit, Council Tax Reduction, and Disability Premium Income Support.

There are a a great many sources of help. Your local GP is a good place to start because they should know what services exist locally.

Many local boroughs have dementia support teams. 85

The Alzheimer's Society can provide a great deal of information that is well written and easy to understand. Many areas have Alzheimer's Society support groups.

Other voluntary organisations such as the Rare Dementia Support and Lewy Body Society can provide information. Admiral Nurses (nurses attached to local health providers but trained by a charity called Dementia UK) can provide help, advocacy and practical support to carers of people with dementia.

There are now several books for people with dementia and their carers. See Chapter 10, Useful Information for contact details of some of the major organisations that produce literature.

Practical help

The need for help in the home and adaptations to the home will change as time goes on. This is why it is so important that the person's needs assessment is done and that a social worker takes responsibility for ensuring that the needs are met and reassessed from time to time. Carers are also entitled to regular assessments. At home, the person with dementia may need:

- help with the housework, shopping and meals on wheels
- safety aids and equipment such as commodes, a laundry service, advice on moving and handling, special clothing, hoists
- home security: a recent development known as

assistive technology, or telecare, can provide imaginative aids to help make the home more safe and secure; these include alarms triggered if a front door is opened or someone falls over, and sensors that sound an alarm if a tap or the gas is left on. Assistive technology also provides some options to tackle the risk of getting lost

- help with bathing, getting up in the morning, dressing and going to bed at night
- help with taking medication
- help with opening and sorting letters and bill payments
- mobility support with activites both indoors and outdoors
- referral for fire assessment by the local fire brigade.

Medical help

Regular visits to the doctor for both the person with dementia and separately for the carer are important.

The person with dementia needs:

- checks with the doctor on a regular basis, ideally every six months
- prompt treatment for other health problems that might occur such as depression or infections
- general health advice about diet and exercise
- regular foot care, checks of vision and hearing, and visits to the dentist.

The carer needs advice on behavioural changes so that they can understand and manage the care of someone with dementia. The carer also needs to look after their own health. A healthy, cheerful carer will make a big difference to the person with dementia with whom they are living or to whom they are close.

Personal support

There are several ways in which both the carer and the person with dementia can receive personal support. All carers are entitled to a carer's assessment. This enables professionals to establish needs and services available to promote well-being and to support carers with their caring needs. The social worker who is responsible for following up the needs assessment and carer's assessment can provide advice and signposting, which might include the areas below.

Taking a break/respite care

Looking after someone with dementia and being looked after can both be emotionally draining. Struggling to manage on one's own can be self-defeating and can make life for the person with dementia more difficult.

It is usually important for both the person with dementia and the carer to have time apart. It is therefore very important for there to be breaks in caring and being cared for. The carer will benefit from being able to socialise with friends, pursue interests or just spend time in the home without having to supervise the person with dementia.

The person with dementia will benefit from being able to socialise with other people and take part in other activities.

Respite can take various forms. The person with dementia might be able to attend a day centre one or more days of the week if it is available locally and the person is willing to go.

It might be possible for someone to come into the home to be with the person with dementia while the carer goes out for an afternoon or evening. Social services may be able to offer longer respite breaks (usually a week or two) in a care home following an assessment of needs.

Someone to talk to

Both carers and people with dementia have described the benefits of talking to other people with similar problems. Support groups exist in many parts of the country. Information about what is available locally can be obtained from your care coordinator or by contacting the Alzheimer's Society or Age UK.

Permanent residential and nursing care

Placement can sometimes strengthen the relationship between people with dementia and their carers, because it allows the carer to be a family member, friend and partner, rather than a caregiver. Professionals will work with carers and people with dementia to exhaust all available options to provide care at home before considering placement. There are a number of reasons for considering placement, such as physical health deterioration, behaviour changes and breakdown of care and support provided in the community. There may come a time when caring for a person with dementia in their own home is getting too difficult or is no longer possible. This will involve discussion among the person with dementia, the carer, the GP or hospital specialist, and the social worker. This might arise if the person with dementia is living alone and becoming a risk to themselves because it is rarely possible to provide 24-hour care to a single person at home, except at great expense.

It might also arise if the person with dementia poses a risk to others. It might arise if the carer living with the person with dementia is physically and mentally frail and cannot manage even with daily help and respite care.

There are four main types of care setting: sheltered and community supportive housing, extra care sheltered housing, residential and nursing homes. Local authorities or the NHS will assess someone for funding if they are thought to need permanent care and all options for keeping someone at home have been tried. If you need to go into residential care you may have to make a contribution to the cost of your care, which you need to discuss with your social worker.

WHO CAN HELP?
Health and social services
The person with dementia, the carer and the social worker, together with the GP, coordinate the care throughout the illness. The GP will be the main person to look after the health care of the person with dementia and the carer.

For a firm diagnosis to be made and advice to be given on further treatment and management, the GP will often refer the person with dementia and the carer to a specialist. This is a free service.

The specialist might be:

- an old age psychiatrist (a doctor specialising in the mental disorders of old age)
- a neurologist (a specialist in diseases of the nervous system)
- a geriatrician (a specialist in medical diseases of older people).

Exactly which specialist someone is referred to will depend on:

- their age
- what symptoms they have
- what services are available locally.

Sometimes it may be necessary for a person to see more than one specialist; for example, a neurologist may ask an old age psychiatrist for a second opinion if symptoms of depression are present.

If the specialist is the old age psychiatrist, they will be part of a community mental health team that often includes social workers, psychologists, occupational therapists and specialist nurses. As the illness progresses, free support and advice may be given by one or more of the members of this team. The other specialists do not generally have a back-up team.

The specialist or the GP can refer to social services for help with bathing and dressing, to the podiatrist/chiropodist for foot care and to the continence adviser.

The occupational therapist can advise on ways of helping someone to maintain their skills and independence for as long as possible. They can also advise on aids in the person's home.

The social worker can organise breaks and respite from caring or being cared for. This can be provided by a number of different agencies – voluntary, private or state – and might have to be paid for.

The social worker will discuss with the person with dementia and the carer what might be most helpful and as time goes on these needs might change. There are a number of possibilities adapted to the particular needs of the person with dementia and the carer, changing with time and local availability, and which might have to be paid for. These are:

- sitters at home to allow a carer to go out for a few hours, an evening, a weekend
- paid carers or volunteers to go out with a person with dementia
- day care organised either by social services or by a voluntary organisation, such as the Alzheimer's Society or Age UK, depending on what is available locally. A person with dementia should be able to go for an agreed number of days a week. Transport is usually arranged by the agency running the day centre
- short-term residential care for a weekend or one or more weeks to allow a carer to go on holiday or just have time on their own at home. This can be provided by social services or by the voluntary or private sector, depending on what is available locally
- permanent residential or nursing home care: this can be arranged with the help of a social worker if the criteria for residential care are met. It is advisable to look at a number of homes. Choice will depend on an assessment of the person with dementia and matching the needs of the person with those that can be met by the home. The choice of home will also depend on the costs of care.

Professionals involved in dementia care

- General practitioners – assessment, diagnosis, care and support
- Psychiatrist – specialist diagnosis and treatment
- Neurologist – specialist diagnosis, rare kinds of dementia
- Occupational therapist – maintainance of independence, aids
- Physiotherapist – assessment of and improvements to mobility
- Community nurse – information, support, monitoring progress
- Admiral nurse – counselling and support for carers
- Social worker – advice on benefits, respite, care homes
- Psychologist – specialist memory tests, analysing behaviours
- Speech and language therapist – improving communication, swallowing problems

THE ALZHEIMER'S SOCIETY

The Alzheimer's Society is dedicated to supporting people with all types of dementias and their families and provides:

- information on all the dementias
- practical and emotional help such as helplines and support groups
- legal and financial advice
- training for carers
- services such as respite care.

Going online[1] is one of the easiest ways of obtaining information. However, if either the person with dementia or the carer has an urgent question, they are strongly advised to telephone the Alzheimer's Society national helpline on 0300 222 1122.

An online forum called Talking Point[2] can be accessed on the Alzheimer's Society website. This is available 24 hours a day and allows you to ask questions, respond to queries from others and participate in discussion.

Joining the Alzheimer's Society and receiving the newsletter help people to keep in touch with news and practical advice.

Other voluntary organisations

You may find really good sources of information and support from a number of local and national organisations, including:

---

1   www.alzheimers.org.uk

2   www.alzheimers.org.uk/talkingpoint/site/index.php www.alzheimers.org.uk/info/20013/talking_point_-_our_online_forum

- Carers UK
- Carers Trust
- Dementia UK
- Age UK
- Citizens Advice – can provide free advice on benefits
- local social services department.

You can find their contact details at the end of this book.

Key points
- People with dementia, and people who look after them, will need information, practical help, medical care and personal support; don't go it alone
- Every carer is entitled to a free needs assessment from the local social services department; ask for it
- Use the Alzheimer's Society; it is there to help you
- It's useful to have a named person to contact for help and advice

6
Living with Dementia

This chapter includes tips for people with dementia and for their carers.

TIPS FOR THE PERSON WITH DEMENTIA

Over the last ten years, more people with dementia have been diagnosed earlier. This has meant that it has been possible to talk to people in the early stages and learn from them what it is like to have the condition.

Not so long ago it was thought impossible that people with dementia could contribute to an understanding of their predicament. Now we have learned a whole range of emotional reactions that they experience from them.

They may be angry: 'Why me?' They may be fearful: 'How will I cope?' 'How will my family cope?' They may feel sad and despairing: 'What is the point of going on?' They may feel alone.

General tips

Here are some tips for people with dementia from people with dementia themselves. If your memory is not as good as it used to be you might find it helpful to:

- keep a diary
- hang a whiteboard in the kitchen showing your weekly timetable and reminders of things that you need to do
- put labels on doors and drawers to remind you where things are kept
- keep a list of telephone numbers with names by the phone
- have a newspaper delivered each day; reading this will help to keep your brain active and remind you of the date
- put things like keys always in the same place to increase the chance of finding them each time you look for them
- tell your family that you do not mind being reminded about things that you need to know
- watch that you do not get depressed. Talk to your friends and family and try to stay as active as possible. Keep up your interests and your friends, and don't be afraid to ask for support. It may be useful to join a group of other people with dementia, which the Alzheimer's Society can find for you. Sharing feelings and ideas

with other people with dementia can be very supportive. You might also want to help the Alzheimer's Society in its work.

At work

If the diagnosis of dementia has been made and you are still at work, unless you are self-employed, you will probably feel that you should leave your job. You or your employer may agree that it is reasonable for you to continue working. You may be pleasantly surprised how considerate people are if they are involved early on.

It might be possible for you to work fewer hours or stay but in a different role. You need to ensure that people tell you if you are not coping, and you need to feel able to ask for support when you need it.

At the point at which you stop working, make sure that you have secured your full pension rights and also get advice about any benefits to which you might be entitled as early as possible, while you are still able to understand them. If your employer has a human resources department there will be someone to help you. If this is not the case try Citizens Advice.

Make sure that you set up a lasting power of attorney so that your affairs can be dealt with if and when you can no longer take responsibility yourself (see below). When you do stop working, try to make sure that you find things to occupy you. Keeping busy, involved and interested is important.

Driving

Dementia can affect people's ability to drive safely. They may feel as if they are able to get about on familiar routes without incident. The problem is that, when a hazard arises, the person may not be able to react as quickly or as well as someone without dementia.

Having a diagnosis of dementia does not mean an automatic driving ban. The person must tell the Driver and Vehicle Licensing Agency (DVLA) and insurance company when they are diagnosed with dementia.

The person is advised not to drive while waiting for the decision from the DVLA. The DVLA may then seek a medical report from the doctor, and may decide to allow the person to continue driving, or offer another driving test. The driving test includes office-based tests and a road test with an experienced examiner.

Sometimes the DVLA will revoke the driving licence. It is not possible to hold a LGV (Large Goods Vehicle) licence or PCV (Public Carriage Vehicle) licence if you have dementia. It is important to be open and honest with the DVLA and the insurance company.

Use of public transport or taxis and walking are probably all safer alternatives.

Everyone has a responsibility to avoid harm not just to themselves but also to the general public. Driving ability usually deteriorates in the 70s and 80s anyway, but this is much more the case in people with dementia so the best advice is to consider stopping driving once you have been given a definite diagnosis of dementia.

FINANCIAL AFFAIRS
General advice

You might need to consult a solicitor about some of the things mentioned here. Make paying bills as simple as possible by getting these paid through the bank on standing orders. Setting up a joint account with a partner may make day-to-day money management easier.

Make sure that you receive all the benefits to which you are entitled. You will be able to obtain this information through the Alzheimer's Society helpline (see Chapter 10, Useful Information).

Make a will

Most people in the UK don't have a will. Dying intestate (without a will) can cause problems for the bereaved family and may mean that assets are left to the wrong people. Writing a will is usually straightforward.

It is probably best to consult a solicitor if you have already been given a diagnosis of dementia. It is still possible for someone with dementia to write a valid will provided that they have 'testamentary capacity'. This means that the person knows:

- the purpose of a will
- what effect the will has (for example, giving money to named people after your death)
- the people who may have a claim on the estate
- roughly how much the estate is worth.

101

The person writing the will must also not have a mental condition that affects their judgement. This does not mean that someone with dementia cannot write a will, but, for example, if someone believes that their son is an imposter and writes him out of the will, that will is not valid.

If in doubt, and certainly where the will is likely to be contentious or challenged, it is a good idea to arrange for a doctor who specialises in mental capacity to assess whether the person has the capacity to make a will. A solicitor should be able to organise this.

Making decisions

As dementia progresses, people are less able to make decisions for themselves. However, in the early stages, many people can make these decisions and influence their lives and care later on.

To be able to make decisions about care, people must have 'mental capacity'. This means that they can: understand and retain information given to them about the issue being decided (for example, a course of treatment or move to a residential home) and the alternative ways of dealing with that issue; weigh this information in the balance and tell someone what they have decided.

If you don't have mental capacity, people caring for you (doctors, nurses, social workers and so on) will have to make decisions on your behalf. There are a number of ways you can make sure your wishes are taken into account in the future if you can no longer make decisions at that time. The earlier you take these steps the better, as you will need to have capacity to put them into place.

It is possible to set up a lasting power of attorney (LPA) (continuing power of attorney in Scotland). There are two types of LPA:

1. A health and welfare lasting power of attorney allows you to nominate one or more people you trust to make decisions about your care and health matters if you are no longer able to do so.
2. A finance and property lasting power of attorney allows you to nominate one or more people to make decisions about your financial affairs.

The person or people you appoint as your attorneys have considerable power and authority so it is best to choose people whom know you well and can trust. Your nominated attorney(s) must take into account what your wishes would have been and must at all times act in your best interests.

You can only complete an LPA if you have capacity to do so. The forms are fairly simple to complete and include an assessment of your capacity at the time you sign the form. This section does not need to be signed by a professional but if you have a diagnosis of dementia it is probably good to get a doctor to sign the mental capacity section of the form.

103

You do not need to go to a solicitor to complete LPA forms – the forms are available from the Office of the Public Guardian. There is a cost (currently £82) for registering these but having LPAs can save considerable costs and heartache later.

You can appoint more than one attorney if you wish, and the welfare attorney and finance attorney can be different people. When completing the form, you can make statements on what you would like to happen (or not happen). When you complete the forms, an independent person (either someone who knows you well or a professional such as a doctor) needs to sign the application stating that you have capacity and are completing the form voluntarily.

LPAs are the best way of ensuring that decisions can be made for you, and they enable someone you trust to look after your finances for you and/or oversee your personal and social care should the time come that you are not able to do this.

If you don't have capacity, people making decisions on your behalf need to decide what is in your best interests. If you have not appointed a welfare attorney, a relative should be consulted about major decisions about care (for example, going into a nursing home) but their opinion is not binding without an LPA.

If there is no one who can do this for you, your social worker will organise for you to have an independent mental capacity advocate (IMCA).

IMCAs are there to help if a serious decision, such

as moving into residential care, needs to be made for you. The IMCA is an independent person who has completed IMCA training and has a background of relevant experience. The role of the IMCA is to support and represent the needs of the person with dementia and do their best to ensure that the right decision is made on that person's behalf.

Advance decisions on treatment

An advance decision allows you to state what treatments you do not wish to receive in the future if you lose mental capacity. It also allows you to communicate your views on issues such as the sanctity of life. The decisions that you may wish to make include whether you would want to die at home or in hospital and whether you would want resuscitation if your heart stops.

When you have written an advance decision, doctors have to follow your wishes if you decline a treatment, but you cannot force them to treat you if this goes against their professional judgement. For example, you can say you don't want antibiotics if you get a chest infection, but you cannot ask doctors to help hasten your death by giving morphine.

A suggested form for setting out an advance decision can be obtained from the Alzheimer's Society. It is important to give a copy to your GP and to your close family, friends or next of kin.

Court of Protection and deputyship

In cases where someone has not appointed a financial power of attorney the local authority may apply for deputyship. This means that the local authority will pay someone's bills and look after their money. If a person has significant assets (for example, property) the Court of Protection may be asked to appoint a deputy who can take over running the person's financial affairs. This could be a relative, a solicitor or an accountant. The family or social worker can apply and a doctor will need to state that a person does not have the capacity to manage their finances.

The Court can be asked to make judgements in cases of complex treatment and welfare decisions (for example, stopping treatment or moving home) in the absence of a welfare attorney.

Further information can be found at the website of the Office of the Public Guardian.[3]

Best interests decisions

In situations where someone does not have mental capacity to make a decision, then the people caring for them have to decide what is in the person's best interests. This applies to all walks of care, including doctors deciding about giving medicine, a care worker deciding on whether to bathe someone and a social worker deciding on whether to place someone in care.

3   www.gov.uk/government/organisations/office-of-the-public-guardian

Decisions vary in complexity and impact. As a rule of thumb, the greater the impact the more people should be consulted. So, for example, a residential carer deciding to cut long toe nails does not need a big discussion. However, deciding to move someone from their home to residential care should involve relatives (or an IMCA), professionals involved in the care such as the occupational therapist, GP or psychiatrist, and the social worker. People making decisions should also consult the person involved, even if they do not have capacity, and must review any advance decisions that have been made. For some big decisions, the Court of Protection can be asked to make the decision.

TIPS FOR THE CARER

Liz, who looks after her husband, says it all:

> My husband first showed symptoms of dementia some years ago. My great difficulty then was getting the professionals to *listen* to me – he presented so well, and was very good at 'covering up'. Now, I know that my quality of life is important and is directly linked with my husband's. When I am exhausted, depressed, emotionally drained, suppressing my irritation and not able to respond in the usual way to verbal abuse and false accusations, I find it very difficult to be patient, tolerant and understanding. I now am very fortunate as my husband goes in for respite care every six weeks for one to two

weeks, and this gives me the chance to sleep, relax
and do the things I am unable to do as a result of
my husband's condition. He has changed from a
confident, capable, outgoing person to a nervous,
frightened, agitated man who no longer reads, enjoys
television or socialises, and scarcely allows me out of
his sight.

Life for the carer can be exhausting. People with
dementia have increasing difficulty carrying out the
activities of daily living without support from their
carers. Life seems to slow down because everything
takes so much longer.

People with dementia may not want to be helped
with some of the more private tasks and may become
very difficult without being able to explain why.
Behaviour can become an embarrassment so that the
carer is ashamed to invite friends home or to go out
with the person. This means that carers are in danger
of becoming isolated and lonely. The person with
dementia might sleep poorly and get mixed up between
day and night, with the result that the carer gets very
tired. The carer may get very sad that they have lost the
person they once knew.

All these emotions can make carers depressed,
angry and irritable, and react impatiently and
aggressively to the person with whom they are living
and for whom they are caring. This can make the
carers feel guilty and even more so if occasionally

they feel that they can no longer cope and want to put the person with dementia into a home. Carers may worry about all the financial implications of caring for someone with a chronic illness.

All these emotions are bound to occur to a lesser or greater extent but they can be substantially reduced with the appropriate advice, information and support. Living with and caring for a person with dementia is challenging.

Here are some general guidelines and tips for carers that other carers have found helpful.

Tips on dealing with toileting and incontinence

The person with dementia may lose the ability to recognise when to go to the toilet, where the toilet is or what to do when in the toilet. The following are some suggestions that other carers have found helpful:

- Remind the person to go to the toilet at regular intervals and always before bedtime or before going out.
- Make sure that the toilet is easy to find, well lit and warm, and leave the door open.
- Make sure that clothing is easy to remove.
- Limit drinks before bedtime or before going out.
- Provide a bottle or commode by the side of the bed.
- Ask the GP to put you in touch with a continence adviser who might be helpful about

109

the use of pads and waterproof covers for the chair and bed.

Tips on dealing with washing and bathing

The person with dementia may forget to wash and no longer recognise the need. Here are some tips:

- Try to establish and maintain a routine.
- Make it fun.
- Respect the person's dignity.
- Think about safety.
- If it is a constant problem, ask the GP to refer you for help from the district nursing service.

Understand what is happening to the person being cared for

People with loss of memory are going to find it difficult to understand what is going on around them, where they are and whom they are with. They might have difficulty expressing themselves or understanding what is being said. They may also be frustrated that they cannot do things for themselves, and become very resistant. Their behaviour might vary from day to day and sometimes within a day – this is the nature of the illness.

It is important for the carer to understand and try to remember that these difficulties are part of the brain disease and not the fault of the person with dementia.

Try to find out as much as possible about dementia and how it is affecting the person for whom you are caring. Your personal knowledge of the person with dementia will often mean that you can understand why they are behaving in the way that they are when this is impossible or at least difficult for professionals.

Keep things normal

Try to keep life going as it has always been for as long as possible. Having a daily routine is helpful but there is a need to be flexible. Keep doing all the things that you have always enjoyed together and seeing friends and family.

Try to consult and involve the person in all decisions, large or small, at all times. This will ensure that their self-esteem is maintained for as long as possible.

Retain the person's independence

It is important that people with dementia continue to carry out the tasks of which they are capable of as long as possible. Everything might take longer and sometimes they may need prompting.

It is often helpful to simplify the tasks, for example laying the clothes on the bed in such a way that the person is assisted to remember in what order to put them on. This allows the person affected to retain a sense of self and dignity.

Encourage activities that a person with dementia has always been interested in doing but remember that 111 with the progression of the illness these interests might change, and you need to pick this up early so as not to cause upset.

It is important that while still able, the person with dementia should be able to go out on their own if they want to. You should make sure the person is carrying some identification, including name and address and the mobile telephone number of a relative or friend. It may be possible to arrange with some of the local shops frequented by the person that they will provide what is asked for and you will settle up afterwards.

Avoid confrontation

Try not to argue when, for example, a person can see no reason for having a bath or changing clothes, or accuses you or someone else of taking their money when they cannot find something. Walk away briefly or think of a distraction and try later.

Avoid crises

When planning to go out, leave enough time so that there is no rush. Remember that unfamiliar places and people will be very confusing. Prepare for these situations by talking and going over things many times beforehand.

Try to anticipate what might happen from what you have already learned. You are the expert because you know the person for whom you are caring better than anyone else.

Try to have a laugh

Life is not easy but the more relaxed you are the better. If you can have a laugh with the person for whom you are caring you will both find it easier to cope.

Lots of hugs can be very reassuring provided, of course, that the person for whom you are caring finds this acceptable.

Make sure that your home is as safe as possible

A confused person is more at risk of accidents simply because they are not paying enough attention due to problems with concentration.

Try to ensure that there are no loose rugs or mats around and that there are handrails up the stairs and in the bathroom. Make sure that slippers fit snugly to reduce the likelihood of falls.

Gas needs to be switched off at the mains if you go out and leave the person for whom you are caring alone. Don't leave matches around.

General health

Regular exercise such as a daily walk and a good diet are essential. The longer the person is fully mobile and physically healthy and cheerful the easier for you and therefore for them.

Take particular care over any drugs taken, supervise them and try to know what each drug is for. Question the doctor if you are not sure about any aspect of medication and if they do not appear to be having 113 any effect. Ask whether any of the drugs can be stopped – the fewer drugs the better.

Make sure that you arrange for the person for whom you are caring to have regular checks of vision, hearing, feet and teeth. Seek advice from the doctor if the person shows symptoms or signs of any physical problems.

Make meal times pleasurable

We all enjoy eating and drinking. Try to involve the person with whom you are living in the planning and preparing of meals and then allow enough time to enjoy it together with a glass of beer or wine, if that is what you have always enjoyed.

Remembering the types of food that the person always used to enjoy can be helpful in deciding what would give most pleasure.

It is important to try to encourage the person to be as independent as possible, so, for example, when the person has difficulty with cutlery, you could offer finger foods more often.

Communication with the person with dementia

Try to gain the person's attention before speaking and remember to speak slowly, clearly and at eye level. Listen and observe carefully. Be prepared to repeat things many times.

Remember that your body language also conveys how you are feeling and will be picked up by the person for whom you are caring.

Try not to ask questions that you think the person with dementia is unlikely to be able to answer or only answer with difficulty as this can cause distress for the person with dementia and can be very frustrating for the carer. For example, if you are expecting a visit from an old friend, don't ask the person what they can remember about the visitor. Assume they cannot remember and talk about the person yourself in some detail. Another example is to try not to ask questions about photos you might spend time looking at together. Assume the person will not recognise the photos and talk about them yourself. Sometimes that sparks a memory and the person might be able to contribute to the conversation.

Telling children and grandchildren about the person with dementia

It is important that children and grandchildren understand about dementia and learn to accept that this is an illness and that they can still give a great deal of pleasure to their parent or grandparent. If children are at school, they will then be able to talk about it to their teachers and friends, and this will mean that they do not feel embarrassed when inviting friends home.

Memory aids

It is helpful to write important things down on a calendar or board in a place that is frequently used. This is useful for things such as plans for the day or remembering the names of people who might be visiting. It is useful to have telephone numbers and names of people with whom one is in regular contact near the telephone. In addition:

- have a clock with clear numbers
- label doors
- have photos of family members around
- when visitors or family come, repeatedly mention their names and who they are.

Communication with the doctor

A good and positive relationship with your doctor and members of the mental health team can make all the difference to how supported you and the person for whom you are caring feel. This will mean working out how best to achieve it. It is really worthwhile to try to ensure that there is a named person in the general practice, the mental health team or the local branch of the Alzheimer Society whom you can talk to easily, as and when problems and questions arise, and who really knows you and the person with dementia. You should have the contact details of this person.

Going to the doctor on a regular basis is important. It does not need to be often. Making the next appointment after each visit is a good idea. It is helpful to come to each visit with some prepared notes on, for example, the patient's general health, changes in the symptoms or behaviour of the person for whom you are caring, side effects of medicines, your own health (see below) and help needed.

When you visit don't be afraid to ask if you do not understand something or want the doctor to repeat something that you have been told. Take notes of what has been said and then you can go over it afterwards.

Look after your own physical and mental health

This is as important as the health of the person for whom you are caring. It is all too easy to neglect your own diet and forget to take exercise when you are busy and exhausted. It is also easy to ignore health problems of your own and not take time to go to the doctor if you need to (see Chapter 5).

Key points
- If you have dementia, try lots of different memory aids; you may find one that suits you and combats the effects of the disease
- If you care for someone with dementia, make sure that you look after your own health and needs
- There are many sources of help and support available – use them
- It is possible for people with dementia to have a good quality of life

7
Future Prospects

The number of people with dementia is increasing. Currently there are about 750,000 people in the UK with various stages of dementia; this will rise to about 1 million by 2030. The main reason for this rise is that people are living longer and people born in the baby boom years are reaching an age where dementia is likely. In 2012, the estimated cost of dementia care in the UK was £23 billion. The bulk of this was the cost of informal (unpaid) care and accommodation.

Despite this, there has been relatively little research into dementia. For every pound spent on cancer research, eight pence is spent on research into dementia.

BETTER DIAGNOSES

A high proportion of people with early dementia are not seen by a doctor until they have had the condition for some time, often years rather than months. Many never receive a diagnosis. This needs to change in the future. This can happen only if there is a further increase in public awareness and a reduction in the stigma associated with the diagnosis.

When people who come with early signs of the condition are assessed, the capacity of doctors to make an accurate diagnosis depends largely on the history provided by the person and their family or friends. Brain scans, memory tests, brain-wave traces and other tests can help with the diagnosis but there is no definitive test for dementia and nothing is as good as a good clinical history.

In the early stages of dementia, it can be impossible to tell for sure whether someone actually has dementia or just the minor memory problems that we all get with advancing age. Developing more accurate tests, especially if they can diagnose dementia very early, is important. More accurate and earlier diagnosis will mean that people can receive treatments more quickly and have more time to maximise the quality of life. Amyloid PET scanning holds real promise here but needs to become more widespread.

Some people have a reversible dementia due to a treatable condition such as an underactive thyroid gland or a vitamin deficiency. Although relatively rare, it is important that doctors recognise when a dementia is treatable so that the cause can be treated. At the moment, about one third of people with dementia do not receive a proper diagnosis so these correctable causes may be missed. All people who develop memory difficulties or problems with thinking should be seen by a doctor to check whether the cause is reversible.

At present, doctors can reliably tell what type of dementia (for example, vascular dementia or Alzheimer's disease) a person has about 80 per cent of the time, based mainly on the history and brain scan. As better treatments emerge for specific types of dementia, the accuracy of telling what type of dementia someone has will become very important, so better tests are needed to distinguish the causes. New and promising developments to aid diagnosis are in the pipeline. Scientists are looking at whether blood tests or tests on the fluid surrounding the spine can help diagnose Alzheimer's disease.

BETTER STANDARDS OF CARE

Most people with dementia are looked after at home, but about a third are looked after in residential homes. If they are living at home, the quality of care that people receive will depend on a range of factors, in particular on whether their carers are well informed about the condition and its course, and how much help and support they get from other members of the family, professionals and the local authority.

At the present time, professional help and support by local services are very variable. Carers are often poorly informed and this needs to change, so that all carers have easy access to the information that they need from the sources that we have already cited.

Many people with dementia will eventually need care in residential homes. Again, the quality of such homes is currently very variable and, in some places, deplorably low. It is vital that people who look after individuals with dementia are properly trained, valued in society and adequately rewarded, and have a career path. Expectations of the standards of care and support for people living at home and in care homes need to rise – something the Care Quality Commission is working on in England.

In the future, it is likely that much greater effort will be made to involve people with dementia in making decisions involving their care than has been the case in the past. Until very recently it has been assumed that it is not really worthwhile to try to find out what such people would like to happen, so professionals and sometimes even family members have not bothered to ask them.

With earlier diagnosis, many more people with dementia are able to take part in decision making. The 2005 Mental Capacity Act makes it compulsory for carers and professionals to consult people with dementia before decisions are taken across a whole range of situations.

TREATMENTS AND CURES

Up to now, dementia has not been seen as a priority for research but this is changing. Also, because scientists have not worked out precisely what causes the many different types of dementia it is difficult to work out what may be a useful treatment.

It seems that almost every week there is some story in the press about a new 'miracle cure'. These stories are nearly always misleading. Although there are many treatments being investigated, these are mainly aimed at helping symptoms of dementia. We are probably many years away from a cure. Sadly, most promising new treatments being developed have not shown to be effective and we are a long way from finding a cure.

Most of the current research is on Alzheimer's disease. As more is understood about how Alzheimer's disease develops, scientists are developing drugs that tackle the disease at different stages.

TREATMENTS FOR BEHAVIOUR PROBLEMS

At least as important as drug treatments for memory are treatments for the behaviour problems occurring in this condition, because often this is the most problematic area for both people with dementia and their carers.

There has been far too much dependence on drugs to manage these problems in the past. In the future, there needs to be much greater emphasis on developing understanding of the problem in the light of the individual's life story and personality.

Key points

In the future:

- the numbers of people with dementia will increase
- greater awareness of the condition and a reduction in stigma may lead to more frequent early diagnosis
- people with dementia should be consulted about decisions involving their care
- although there is no immediate prospect of a cure, new diagnostic techniques and treatments are being developed

8
Questions and Answers

What is dementia?

Dementia is the general name used to describe the large number of disorders of the brain where there is a progressive deterioration of brain function such as memory, thinking, language and personality.

Is Alzheimer's disease different from dementia?

No. It is not different. Alzheimer's disease is one kind of dementia. It is the most common form but there are many other less common types.

How is a diagnosis of dementia made?

There is no specific test. The diagnosis is usually made either by the GP or by a specialist (psychiatrist or neurologist) who will take a history and ask about the symptoms from both the person with the problem and a close family member or close friend. The history, together with some blood tests, memory tests and possibly a brain scan, will normally make it possible to arrive at a diagnosis.

Can I be tested to see if I have dementia?

A diagnosis is reached in the ways described in answer to the previous question. If you are worried that you have dementia, see your doctor to discuss your concerns.

What causes dementia?

The basic cause of all types of dementia is damage to the nerve cells in the brain. The changes in the brain depend on the type of dementia, of which the most common is Alzheimer's disease and the second, but less common, type is vascular dementia.

In Alzheimer's disease one can see characteristic abnormalities in the brain called plaques and tangles. In vascular dementia there is disease of the blood vessels and evidence of areas of dead tissue in the brain due to mini-strokes. However, nearly all people with Alzheimer's disease also have some degree of vascular disease. Pure vascular dementia is a much less common type of dementia.

Then there is the question of why some people develop these diseases and others don't. An individual's gene structure (inherited factors) may make them more vulnerable to developing Alzheimer's disease, but there are very few people for whom genes are the only important cause of this condition.

125

There must also be a number of environmental and lifestyle causes of Alzheimer's disease, but it has not so far proved possible to identify conclusively what they are.

How will I know if I am developing dementia?

It has become very common for people to think that they have a dementia when they forget something. This is because there is so much greater awareness of dementia that people talk and worry about it more. You sometimes hear people jokingly saying that they must be getting 'Alzheimer's' when they forget someone's name or telephone number or a film that they have seen recently.

In some cases, a person developing dementia is the first to become aware of a memory problem, but usually it is the people around them who are the first to notice. So if you think that you may be susceptible, you should be prepared to ask people close to you, or who work with you, if and when they notice a problem with your memory to tell you about it.

Will I get dementia?

We know that the chance of getting dementia increases with age, although we do not know why this is. If there are people in your family who have definitely developed dementia as they have got older, your chance of developing it is slightly greater if you also live to an old age.

What can I do if I do get dementia?

Don't lose heart. Join the Alzheimer's Society. Find out everything that you can about it. Find other people with dementia to talk to. Don't be afraid to tell people to whom you are close that you have dementia. Try your best to lead as normal a life as possible (for further tips, see Chapter 6, Living with Dementia).

How can I prevent dementia?

Many people with dementia also have evidence of blood vessel changes. Clots in the blood vessels leading to the heart give rise to heart attacks. Clots in the vessels to the brain can lead to strokes. Large or multiple small strokes can lead to dementia.

Anything that can reduce the formation of blood clots definitely reduces the risk of heart attacks and strokes. So what is good for the heart is good for the brain. We recommend the following:

- Get your hearing tested.
- Maintain a healthy diet – low in saturated fat.
- Don't smoke.
- Consume alcohol in moderation.
- Take regular exercise both physical and mental.
- Don't get overweight.
- Control diabetes if present.
- Control high blood pressure if present.
- Keep your mind busy.

127

There is no guarantee that you will not get dementia if you pay attention to all these factors, but they are good for you anyway!

I have been told that I have dementia. Is there a cure?

No. At this point in time there is no cure. If you are lucky enough to get a good response to drug treatment then it might appear that you are 'cured' for a while. However, these drugs do not affect the disease process so the symptoms will return sooner or later. If they do not, it is highly likely that you did not have the correct diagnosis in the first place.

Are there drugs to stop the dementia getting worse?

Yes. There are drugs that help some people with dementia to function better in their everyday lives, such as donepezil, galantamine and rivastigmine. They do not help everyone who takes them. We are not yet able to predict who will respond positively.

If a person is helped, the drugs may delay progress of the dementia for about a year but this varies from person to person. In people who have responded to drugs it is important to continue them as any benefits may be lost if the drug is stopped, even years later.

I have been given a diagnosis of dementia. Can I drive?

Possibly, but you (or sometimes your doctor) will need to notify the Driver and Vehicle Licensing Agency (DVLA) and wait for its decision. The DVLA will ask for a medical report and may decide on the basis of this to renew your licence for a year or revoke your licence. Sometimes it may offer a new driving test to reassess your driving ability.

You would be well advised to start adapting to the idea that you will not be able to carry on driving for too much longer, and start using public transport and taxis or allowing other people to drive you.

Where can I get more information about dementia?

The very best source of information is available from the Alzheimer's Society. GPs or specialists who make a diagnosis of dementia should routinely give you the address, telephone number and website of the Alzheimer's Society. The information is available in printed form and on the internet and there is a helpline available to everyone (see Chapter 10, Useful Information).

Are there drug trials in which I can take part?

You should ask your GP or specialist if they are doing any or if there are any trials being done not too far from where you live. This is also a question that the Alzheimer's Society might be able to help with.

I care for my husband who has dementia. Who can I ring when I get desperate?

We hope that you will have enough support to make sure that you never get desperate. However, there might well be times when you feel that way. You need to have a list of numbers you can ring by your phone. These should include:

- your GP
- the named person in the community mental health team whom you have been seeing
- a friend from your support group with whom you have this arrangement
- the helpline of the Alzheimer's Society or Dementia UK
- a neighbour or relative with whom you have this arrangement.

My mother is showing worrying signs of memory loss but refuses to go to the doctor and denies that she has a problem. What shall I do?

Try making an appointment yourself with your mother's GP and tell them about your concerns. A good GP will listen to you and then probably recommend that you tell your mother that you have been to see the GP and that the GP would like to come and take your mother's blood pressure and do a routine check-up. It is important that you arrange to be present when the doctor visits.

My father has dementia. My mother is struggling with everything that she has to do. They adamantly refuse help from outside services. What shall I do?

Do try to persuade your mother to talk with social services. If there is a problem with money you might be able to help by finding out about and then explaining to your parents the Attendance Allowance. This is intended to buy extra help, so, if your father qualifies, try to persuade your parents to use or allow you to use the money for this purpose. Or you might need to pay for it yourself initially.

You might need to spend time finding someone who can help with the washing, cleaning and shopping. Try to be present the first few times that this person comes to help.

How are we going to choose the right home for my mother who has dementia?

You will want to talk this over with your social worker who might have some homes to suggest to you. The Alzheimer's Society helpline or the Elderly Accommodation Council (see Chapter 10, Useful Information) might be able to give you a list. However, lists will only be able to give you names.

If you have access to the internet (you can get this in a public library), you can look up different homes and find the most recent Care Quality Commission report. If you do not have access to the internet, you can ring the customer helpline for the Care Quality Commission (see Chapter 10, Useful Information) and ask for details of recent reports of homes in which you might be interested. Then you will need to visit some of the homes that you have chosen and ask some questions.

The Alzheimer's Society has a good factsheet on the sort of questions that you might want to ask when you visit a home. You might find it useful to organise for your mother to spend a day or even a respite admission in a home that you have found to see how she responds. This may be a lengthy process but it is well worth taking time over it.

My mother who has dementia and lives on her own cannot cope at home now. What is available for her?

There are four main types of care settings.

Sheltered and community supportive housing

In sheltered (or community supportive) accommodation there is often a scheme manager or locally based team that will regularly call on and check residents to make sure that they are okay. Residents will also be provided with an alarm system so that they can call for help in an emergency at any time of the day or night.

If you move to a specialist sheltered or supported accommodation scheme you will have to pay rent on your flat, and sometimes an additional service charge which covers the services of the scheme manager, and general maintenance. If you are eligible for Housing Benefit then you will be able to claim this towards the cost of your rent. Sheltered and community supportive schemes are usually owned by your local council, or run by a housing association on behalf of the council. Tenants will have a secure tenancy with the same rights as other council tenants. You will usually have to complete the same application form as you would for any council housing, but you should tell them that you are particularly interested in sheltered and supported accommodation.

Extra care sheltered housing

Extra care is like sheltered housing but with far more support on site. To be considered for extra care housing you will need to have had a community care assessment from your local council. A social worker will then be able to look at your needs and help you to decide whether extra care housing is the best option for you based on the amount of support that you need.

Depending on your financial situation, you may be able to claim Housing Benefit towards the rent for your extra-care flat. You may also need to pay

133

towards the cost of the support that you receive, just as you would if you were receiving this support in your previous home.

Residential homes
Residential homes provide support for people who don't have complex needs. The staff in care homes will generally be trained care workers rather than trained nurses, but should have all the skills required to provide the necessary support.

Nursing homes
Nursing homes support people with higher, more complex levels of need. Some of the staff on duty at any time will be trained nurses working alongside the trained care workers. Nursing homes cost more because they provide a greater level of support. You will want to be sure that you are choosing a home for your mother with the right level of support for her.

Some people with very severe behavioural problems may qualify for NHS continuing care (see below).

Who will pay for my mother's care home?
Almost all people needing support in a care home will be expected to pay something towards the costs of their accommodation and personal care. How much they pay will depend on their financial situation. Your mother may be eligible for financial support from the council to pay for the cost of a care home. This will

depend on whether the council agrees that your
mother needs such a high level of care following an
assessment of her needs, and will also depend on
an assessment of her financial circumstances to find
out how much, if any, the council should be paying
towards the cost of the care. This financial assessment,
or 'means test', is based on nationally set guidelines
and looks at how much income and capital (savings,
assets and property) your mother has. If your mother
has over a certain amount in savings (a figure set by the
government currently at £23,250) she will probably be
required to pay for the full costs of her care for as long
as her savings remain above this amount. If she has
less than this amount in savings, she may be entitled to
financial help.

If she alone owns a property that can be sold, its
value may be taken into account when the council
works out how much she should pay towards her care
home. When the new Care Act came into effect on
1 April 2015 the way in which the council works out
how much she can afford to pay towards the cost of
a care home remained largely unchanged. However,
in some cases the council now has a duty to offer
your mother a deferred payment scheme when she
moves into a care home, meaning that she will not
immediately need to sell her own home in order to pay
for the care home. If your mother lives with your father
and he wishes to remain in the house then the property

is not included in your mother's financial assessment now or in the future.

If your mother is assessed as having nursing needs then she will have a second assessment by the NHS of her registered nursing input needs.

If it is confirmed that she does have nursing needs then the NHS pay the nursing home a flat rate, which at the time of writing is £155.05 per week. This is the amount of money that the NHS will contribute to her care in addition to the money paid by her and the local authority.

In some severe and complex cases, the NHS will cover all the costs. This would be applicable if your mother needs constant nursing care and regular supervision by a hospital specialist because she is very frail or severely mentally ill or exhibiting continuous difficult behaviour.

As the carer of my mother with dementia is she or am I entitled to any benefits?

As a carer you could get £62.70 a week if you care for someone at least 35 hours a week and they get certain benefits. You don't have to be related to, or live with, the person you care for. However, this may affect other benefits that you or your mother receive, so check this out. You won't be paid extra if you care for more than one person.

As the person with dementia, you might be entitled to Personal Independent Payment (PIP) or Attendance

Allowance. If you are eligible for Attendance Allowance, you could get £55.65 or £83.10 a week to help with personal care because you are physically or mentally disabled and you are aged 65 or over. It's paid at two different rates and how much you get depends on the level of care that you need because of your disability.

The Attendance Allowance is for people over the age of 65 and the Disability Living Allowance for people under the age of 65. These benefits are not dependent on income or savings and are tax free.

It is important that you ask advice about this from your social worker, the Alzheimer's Society or your local Citizens Advice service. The Disability Service Centre also has helplines for people with disabilities, including those with dementia, where you can find out more about benefits you may be entitled to (see Chapter 10, Useful Information).

You or your mother may be entitled to a reduction in or exemption from the council tax. Ask your council about this.

My father has dementia and is making mistakes with his money. What should I do about this?

If this has not already been done, probably the most important step is for your father (the donor) to make out a lasting power of attorney (LPA), provided that he still has the capacity to do this (see Chapter 6 Living with Dementia).

This enables a person of his choice (the attorney)

to look after his finances when he can no longer do so. It is the responsibility of the attorney to decide when your father is no longer able to manage his financial affairs. If he has any doubts he can ask a doctor for advice.

You can get the necessary forms free from the Office of the Public Guardian – available on the internet. These forms can look quite complicated and he and you might need help completing them.

You might find it useful to consult a solicitor, although this is not essential. The organisation Solicitors for the Elderly specialises in helping people with all kinds of legal advice, including help with the LPA. This is expensive but it might be a good deal more expensive not to do this properly. It is important to have a completed LPA made out before the person with dementia no longer has the capacity (mental ability) to do this.

If your father wants to set up a power of attorney, an independent person needs to sign a declaration that he understands and agrees to this. This may be a person whom he has known for over two years or a professional such as a doctor.

If this person has any doubt about your father's capacity, you should ask his doctor or local old age psychiatrist to make a capacity assessment. Capacity in this case means that your father is able to understand what the LPA involves and can choose a person he trusts to look after his finances.

There are a number of other practical things that you can do if he agrees, such as making arrangements with his bank to allow him to withdraw only small amounts of money at a time, organising for bills and pensions to be paid direct from the bank, and telling the local shops of his problem. In this way, you can help your father to remain independent for as long as possible without making expensive mistakes.

If your father is no longer able to set up an LPA, you may need to apply to the Court of Protection for financial deputyship. The court may then appoint you to look after his affairs.

I'm worried that my mother's neighbour is regularly taking money from her. My mum is very confused now. What can I do?

In addition to protecting your mother's money as outlined in the question above, this may be a case of financial exploitation. Your local social services has a duty to investigate this using a procedure called safeguarding. You can raise a safegaurding alert by speaking to your mother's social worker or phoning the local social services duty team.

By raising a safeguarding alert, you can ensure that the matter is investigated. Financial exploitation is against the law and the police may investigate this. If you think a crime is being committed it's best to inform the police straight away by calling 101.

Should my wife be told she has Alzheimer's disease?

It is always helpful to tell the person with dementia about their diagnosis. The distress that you feel this might cause may well be lessened by the fact that your wife might already realise that something is wrong. Furthermore, some people are even quite relieved to have a name to give their problem.

My two brothers refuse to acknowledge that my husband has dementia or any problem at all with his memory. I need their support. What can I do?

Try to arrange for your brothers to spend more time with your husband on their own. They will soon realise that something is amiss. Try to arrange for someone from the mental health team to explain to your brothers what is wrong.

My mother who has dementia no longer says anything at all and does not appear to understand anything I say to her. Do you think she might still have some understanding? Can you advise how I should communicate with her?

You should assume that she understands at least part of what you say to her. She will certainly continue to appreciate your company and care. She may still be sensitive to your feelings of love and affection, or sometimes irritation. You need to continue to talk to her and have physical contact with her.

My father has dementia. I am at a loss to know what to talk about with him. I know that the person I pay to be with him when I am out also has this problem. Can you advise?

You will know your father really well. Try to get on to topics that you have heard him talk about many times before. It might mean listening to the same stories over and over again. But the opportunity to speak in this way will give your father a great sense of self-esteem. Memories from early life are often present in people with advanced dementia, and talking about early experiences can be a way in. It is extremely helpful to people who will not know your father so well to have available a simple description of his life in terms of school, work, marriage, family, hobbies and interests. This should include some photographs if possible.

My wife has dementia and has been admitted to hospital for an operation. Do you have any advice?

Try to stay with your wife as much as possible. Your wife may appear more confused because she is in a strange environment. The anaesthetic and operation may also make her temporarily more confused. Speak to the nurse in charge and make sure the staff know about your wife's diagnosis. Many hospitals now encourage people to stay with relatives with dementia (see www.johnscampaign.org.uk).

9
How Your Brain Works

THE CONSCIOUS AND SUBCONSCIOUS

The brain is by far the most complex and sophisticated organ in the body. It enables us to think, remember, move around, speak, interpret vision, sound, smell, taste and touch, and make decisions. These processes are all conscious; in other words, we are aware of these events.

The brain also performs a lot of subconscious tasks of which we are not aware. For example, it controls our vital body systems such as breathing, heart and blood pressure. It also produces various hormones that regulate our metabolism and other body systems.

THE ANATOMY OF THE BRAIN

The healthy adult brain weighs about 1.3 kilograms (about 2 pounds) and is thought to contain about 100 billion nerve cells called neurons. Once we reach adolescence, the brain does not create any new neurons.

The size and structure of these neurons vary depending on the role that they play. For example, neurons responsible for movement are very different to those that interpret vision.

Neurons allow messages to be transmitted between different parts of the brain and to the rest of the body by tiny electrical impulses. Rather than just a big mass of neurons, the brain is highly organised into different areas, which communicate with each other via bundles of neurons called tracts. The result is a web of highly organised connections.

Nerve transmission

Neurons connect to each other through tiny spaces between nerve cells called synapses. Neurons have between 1000 and 10,000 synapses and are constantly communicating with each other by releasing chemicals called neurotransmitters. (You are able to understand what you are reading in this book because nerve cells are firing messages and releasing neurotransmitters.)

When an electrical impulse travels down a neuron, synapses will be activated to release a small amount of neurotransmitter (Figure 9.1). There are many different neurotransmitters with different functions. For example, some neurotransmitters activate the next nerve cell in the chain, whereas others inhibit it.

Whatever their function, all neurons have a similar structure. The centre of the neuron is the nucleus. Typically, several short fibres called dendrites run to the nucleus. These transmit nerve impulses to the

143

centre. A single fibre, called an axon, transmits nerve impulses away from the nucleus.

To stay healthy, the brain requires a lot of oxygen and glucose, which is supplied by large blood vessels (the carotid and vertebral arteries). About a litre of blood (about one fifth of the heart's output) passes through the brain every minute. Any interruption to the blood supply can quickly lead to nerve cell damage.

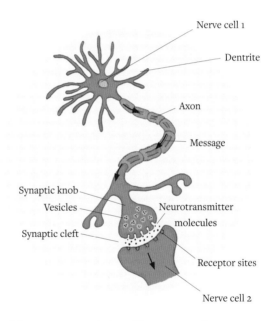

Figure 9.1: Message transmission: Neurotransmitter molecules cross the synaptic cleft and attach to the receptor sites, so passing on the message

FUNCTIONS OF DIFFERENT PARTS OF THE BRAIN

The brain is divided into two main areas: the outer surface is called the cortex (where conscious processes are thought to occur) and the inner part the medulla. Deep within the brain are areas called the midbrain and brain stem. These areas integrate impulses from different parts of the brain and information coming from the rest of the body (rather like a complex telephone exchange) and control our subconscious processes such as blood pressure and heart rate. The cerebellum, located near the back of the brain, helps control movement.

The cortex

The cortex, on the surface of the brain, is divided into different areas, called lobes, which have different functions (Figure 9.2). Although it is probably over-simplifying the brain function somewhat, it is useful to know what lobes are important in different processes in the brain.

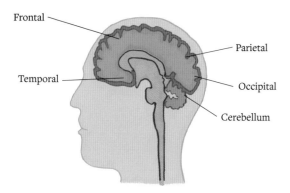

Figure 9.2: Lobes of the brain

Frontal lobes

The frontal lobe (the largest lobe, sitting over the front half of the brain) has many functions, including abstract thinking, planning and making decisions. It is thought to be the area that controls urges and behaviours; some people who have damage to the frontal lobes may become disinhibited and do strange or embarrassing things; others may become unmotivated and apathetic. The back part of the frontal lobe is where voluntary movement is controlled.

Parietal lobe

Behind the frontal lobe is the parietal lobe. This is involved in interpreting touch and hearing, and collects information from other sensory systems (such as vision) to help us integrate different sensations. Damage to the parietal lobe can result in someone not being able to understand sensory inputs.

Temporal lobe

The temporal lobe is tucked underneath the frontal and parietal lobes and is thought to be the main site for memory, but is also involved in hearing and understanding speech. People with damage to the temporal lobe may have great difficulty in remembering things. A part of the temporal lobe called the hippocampus, sometimes regarded as the main seat of memory, is affected early in Alzheimer's disease.

Occipital lobe

At the back of the brain is the occipital lobe, which is the main part of the brain involved in interpretation of vision.

MEMORY

Memory is the process of registering new information, storing it and recalling it when needed. We are constantly laying down new memories.

Scientists have suggested that there are two main types of memory.

Short-term memory

Short-term memory retains a small amount of information (about seven items) for up to 30 seconds. For example, we can often remember a new phone number or car registration number for just long enough to write it down, but if something else happens we quickly forget this information.

Long-term memory

Memories can move from short-term to long-term memory. Memories may move into the long-term memory because we repeat the fact again and again (such as learning lines for a play) or the memory is associated with a strong emotion. For instance, most people can recall incidents that made them very upset or frightened. This is known as flashbulb memory.

Memory can also be classified according to the type of information stored. Procedural memory requires no conscious effort to recall. It often refers to routine things that we do. For example, an experienced car driver would not have to think 'how do I use this?' when they get behind the wheel.

Declarative (or explicit) memory does require conscious effort – if you want to drive to see a friend you need to consciously remember what their address is. Declarative memory is sometimes further divided into semantic and episodic memory.

Semantic memory encodes general facts, not related to a particular time or place or context. Episodic memory is related to a particular context. For example, remembering that someone is your friend would be semantic memory, but recalling that you last saw them when you visited the seaside on a hot Saturday afternoon last summer would be episodic memory.

EFFECT OF DEMENTIAS ON BRAIN STRUCTURE AND FUNCTION

One of the hallmarks of most kinds of dementia is shrinkage of the brain. This is thought to be due to the dying off of some of the nerve cells. In most kinds of dementia, the amount of some chemicals in the brain is reduced, leading to problems with nerve cells communicating with each other.

The loss of nerve cells combined with the loss of chemicals results in symptoms such as loss of memory, change in personality, and difficulties in thinking, planning and language.

Although it may vary from person to person, most people with dementia will develop problems with memory first. The ability to store new memories declines, often subtly at first. Frequently, more recent memories are often lost first in dementia. Memories from childhood may remain well after someone has forgotten recent events.

Key points
- The brain is a complex organ with a highly organised network of 100 billion nerve cells
- Brain cells communicate with each other using chemicals called neurotransmitters
- In dementia, there is a reduction of nerve cells and neurotransmitters

10
Useful Information

USEFUL ADDRESSES

We have included the following organisations because, on preliminary investigation, they may be of use to the reader. However, we do not have first-hand experience of each organisation and so cannot guarantee the organisation's integrity. Readers must therefore exercise their own discretion and judgement when making further enquiries.

Age UK London
Tavis House, 1–6 Tavistock Square, London WC1H 9NA
Helpline: 0800 678 1174
Website: www.ageuk.org.uk
Researches the needs of older people and is involved in policy making. Provides advice on a range of subjects for people aged over 50. Publishes books and offers services via local branches.

Alzheimer's Disease International
64 Great Suffolk Street, London SE1 0BL

Tel: 020 7981 0880
Website: www.alz.co.uk
The global federation of Alzheimer associations around the world.

Alzheimer Scotland – Action on Dementia

160 Dundee Street, Edinburgh EH11 1DQ
Tel: 0131 243 1453
Helpline: 0808 808 3000
Website: www.alzscot.org
Provides advice, support and local services in Scotland for people with dementia and their carers.

Alzheimer's Society

43–44 Crutched Friars, London EC3N 2AE
Tel: 0330 333 0804
Helpline: 0300 222 1122
Website: www.alzheimers.org.uk
UK's leading dementia support and research charity for anyone affected by any form of dementia in England, Wales and Northern Ireland.

The Alzheimer Society of Ireland

Temple Road, Blackrock, Co. Dublin, Ireland
Tel: +353 (0)1 207 3800
Helpline: 1800 341 341
Website: www.alzheimer.ie
The leading dementia specific service provider in Ireland.

Care Quality Commission

CQC National Customer Service Centre, Citygate, Gallowgate, Newcastle upon Tyne NE1 4PA
Tel: 0300 061 6161

Website: www.cqc.org.uk
The official body regulating care homes and agencies that provide nurses or care workers who carry out personal tasks.

Carers Trust

32–36 Loman Street, London SE1 OEH
Tel: 0300 772 9600
Website: www.carers.org
Crossroads care and Princess Royal Trust for Carers have merged to form the Carers Trust. Largest provider of comprehensive support services for carers in the UK. Provides quality information, advice and support services to carers, including young carers. Also has offices in Scotland, Wales and Northern Ireland.

Carers UK

20 Great Dover Street, London SE1 4LX
Tel: 020 7378 4999
Helpline: 0808 808 7777 (Wed, Thurs 10am–12 noon, 2–4pm)
Website: www.carersuk.org
Encourages carers to recognise their own needs. Offers information, advice and support to all people who are unpaid carers looking after others with medical or other problems. Branches organise activities, social events and helplines to help carers.

Citizens Advice

200 Aldersgate Street, London EC1A 4HD
Tel: 0300 023 1231
Website: www.citizensadvice.org.uk
HQ of national charity offering a wide variety of practical, financial and legal advice. Network of local charities

throughout the UK listed in phone books and in *Yellow Pages* under 'Counselling and Advice'.

CJD Support Network

PO Box 346, Market Drayton, Shropshire TF9 4WN
Tel: 01630 673993
Helpline: 0800 085 3527
Website: www.cjdsupport.net
Provides help and support for people with all strains of Creutzfeldt–Jakob disease (CJD), their carers and concerned professionals. Runs a national helpline and can help families in financial need.

Court of Protection

See Office of the Public Guardian.

Dementia UK

2nd Floor, 356 Holloway Road, London N7 6PA
Tel: 020 7697 4160
Helpline: 0800 888 6678
Website: www.dementiauk.org
Focuses on providing specialist dementia nurses (Admiral Nurses) who can offer practical advice, emotional support and skills to families and carers of people with dementia.

Disability Service Centre – gov.uk

Tel: 0345 605 6055
Website: www.gov.uk/disability-benefits-helpline
Advice and information about a claim you've already made for Disability Living Allowance, Attendance Allowance or Personal Independence Payment.

Driver Vehicle and Licensing Agency (DVLA)

Swansea SA6 7JL

Tel (for medical issues): 0300 790 6806

Website: www.dvla.gov.uk

Provides advice about different conditions such as dementia and driving.

Elderly Accommodation Counsel

89 Albert Embankment, London SE1 7TP

Tel: 0800 377 7070

Website: www.eac.org.uk

A source of information on all forms of accommodation for older people.

Huntington's Disease Association

Suite 24, Liverpool Science Park Innovation Centre I,
131 Mount Pleasant, Liverpool L3 5TF

Tel: 0151 331 5444

Website: www.hda.org.uk

Offers support and understanding to anyone affected by Huntington's disease. Has a network of regional care advisers who provide information, workshops and educational services.

Innovations in Dementia

PO Box 616, Exeter EX1 9JB

Tel: 01392 420076

Website: www.innovationsindementia.org.uk

A community interest company involved with people who have dementia. Believes in the human rights and potential of people with dementia and committed to demonstrating how a more positive approach can work in practice.

National Council for Palliative Care

Hospice House, 34–44 Britannia Street, London WC1X 9JG
Tel: 020 7697 1520
Website: www.ncpc.org.uk
Promotes the extension and improvement of palliative care
services for all people with life-threatening and life-limiting
conditions.

National Institute for Health and Care Excellence (NICE)

1st Floor, 10 Spring Gardens, London SW1A 2BU
Tel: 0300 323 0748
Website: www.nice.org.uk
Provides national guidance on the promotion of good health
and the prevention and treatment of ill-health. Patient
information leaflets are available for each piece of guidance
issued.

Office of the Public Guardian

PO Box 16185, Birmingham B2 2WH
Tel: 0300 456 0300
Website: www.gov.uk/government/organisations/office-of-
the-public-guardian
Protects people in England and Wales who may not have the
mental capacity to make certain decisions for themselves,
such as about their health and finance.

Parkinson's UK

National Office, 215 Vauxhall Bridge Road, London SW1V 1EJ
Tel: 020 7931 8080
Helpline: 0808 800 0303
Website: www.parkinsons.org.uk
Provides information and support for people with
Parkinson's disease and their carers.

USEFUL LINKS

BBC
www.bbc.co.uk/health
A helpful website: easy to navigate and offers lots of useful advice and information. Also contains links to other related topics.

Healthtalk.org
www.healthtalkonline.org
Information and support provided by seeing and hearing about people's real-life experiences.

Lewy Body Society
www.lewybody.org
Raises awareness and educates the public, the medical profession and those in health-care decision-making positions about Lewy body disease.

Rare Dementia Support
www.raredementiasupport.org
Runs specialist support services for people living with frontotemporal dementia and other rare dementias.

Solicitors for the Elderly
www.sfe.legal
A national organisation of lawyers, such as solicitors, barristers and legal executives, who are committed to providing and promoting robust, comprehensive and independent legal advice for older people, their families and carers.

Index